GETTING THE MOST FOR YOUR MEDICAL DOLLAR

OTHER BOOKS FROM
THE PEOPLE'S MEDICAL SOCIETY

Allergies: Questions You Have...Answers You Need

Diabetes: Questions You Have...Answers You Need

Exercise and Arthritis: A Guide to Pain-Free Movement

Managed Care Made Easy

Massage Made Easy

Medicare Made Easy

Take This Book to the Gynecologist With You

Take This Book to the Hospital With You

Take This Book to the Pediatrician With You

The Complete Book of Relaxation Techniques

The Parent's Complete Guide to Ear Infections

So You're Going to Be a Mother

Yoga Made Easy

GETTING THE MOST FOR YOUR MEDICAL DOLLAR

By Charles B. Inlander
and
The Staff of the People's Medical Society

People's Medical Society®
Allentown, Pennsylvania

The People's Medical Society is a nonprofit consumer health organization dedicated to the principles of better, more responsive and less expensive medical care. Organized in 1983, the People's Medical Society puts previously unavailable medical information into the hands of consumers so that they can make informed decisions about their own health care.

Membership in the People's Medical Society is $20 a year and includes a subscription to the *People's Medical Society Newsletter.* For information, write to the People's Medical Society, 462 Walnut Street, Allentown, PA 18102, or call 610-770-1670.

This and other People's Medical Society publications are available for quantity purchase at discount. Contact the People's Medical Society for details.

Printed in the United States of America

ISBN 1-882606-41-8 (pbk.)

PART I

THE SAVVY MEDICAL CONSUMER

INTRODUCTION

It takes a savvy consumer to cut through the maze known as the American health-care system. But with the right information, the right attitude and a willingness to be just a little assertive, you can get quality health care at a cost far less than what many of your friends and neighbors pay.

Despite all its virtues, all its miracles and all its victories, our health-care system is fraught with physical and economic dangers. It is a system that even renowned medical experts have labeled "out of control."

There are 42 million Americans without health insurance. Another 30 million people are underinsured—they could not cover their medical bills if confronted with a major illness or a prolonged medical encounter. Corporations that once provided liberal health-care benefits to employees at little or no cost now require employees to pay part of their insurance premiums, deductibles and copayments. Some companies have even cut their benefits. Most have switched to managed-care programs, like health maintenance organizations (HMOs).

The numbers tell the story. In 1996, the United States spent 14.5 percent of its gross national product on health care. That's $1 trillion, or more than three times what we spent on national defense. It also represented a 5 percent increase over the previous year. Overall inflation for the same period was around 3 percent. And while health-care inflation has leveled off for the last several years, analysts predict it will start climbing again as baby boomers reach their 50s and start needing more medical services.

If those numbers don't hit home, try these. The average American household of four spends $14,000 each year for health-care services. This includes out-of-pocket payments to doctors and hospitals, insurance premiums, medical equipment purchases, federal and state taxes used for health care and the cost of health-care benefits built into the goods and services you buy.

Under normal economic circumstances, health-care costs should be going down. Demand is nowhere near the level of supply. Approximately 55 percent of the hospital beds in this country are empty. Every one of America's major cities has a doctor glut—many more doctors than we need in order to provide quality care to consumers. A coronary bypass, a procedure that has increased in frequency by more than 100 percent in the last 10 years, went from an average of $20,000 per procedure in 1980 to close to $50,000 in 1995. Yet in the 1970s, when that particular operation was coming into vogue, medical gurus were promising a dramatic drop in cost as the operation became more commonplace. That's a pretty serious medical misdiagnosis.

Even the quality of American medicine is coming into question. Hospital infections are rampant. One out of 10 people who enter a hospital today can expect to acquire an infection they did not have when they were admitted. That is an almost 100 percent increase in the last decade. Twenty percent of all people who enter a hospital acquire a condition while in the hospital that they did not have before they came. Several studies have shown that up to 40 percent of the people admitted to hospitals are there as a result of something a doctor has done to them.

Americans get the most health care in the world and pay the highest fees for it, yet overall the nation ranks relatively low, compared with other developed countries, in such categories as length of life and infant mortality.

As a result, consumers now are taking a more "buyer beware" attitude about medical services. We are questioning more, saying no to what appear to be useless or unnecessary services, seeking second opinions, using outpatient services and entering wellness and rehabilitation programs.

The federal government, insurers and businesses have implemented programs such as HMOs and other managed-care models that require patients to get preapproval for treatments to ensure that the consumer is getting the right treatment for the condition presented. Medicare beneficiaries are staying fewer days in the hospital than before and are being urged to join cost-saving Medicare HMOs. Insurance companies are encouraging the use of less costly outpatient services. Businesses are telling their employees to use fewer medical services and to use them only when absolutely necessary.

Yet medical inflation continues to outpace general inflation. And even with managed care becoming the predominant form of medical insurance, the number of uninsured continues to rise, the cost of care continues to go up, and the quality of care continues to be questionable. Hospitals are merging with one another to survive, with many moving from nonprofit to for-profit status. Insurers that were once nonprofit are also switching over to for-profit status. They all say it's to compete in this highly competitive market. But the bottom line for you is more cost and uncertain quality. And the bottom line for the hospitals and insurers is bigger profits than ever before.

The change in the health-care system has not only affected consumers, but it's also affected practitioners. Now they must answer to the payer, either a managed-care company, insurer, government or large employer. Until just a few years ago, doctors ruled the roost. They told payers how much a service would cost, and payers forked over the cash. Today payers negotiate fees and payments based on the volume of business they can send a doctor's way. And, despite all their yelling and screaming, doctors and other practitioners are cutting deals, while they still try to deny they are business types.

They talk about caring, healing, touching and compassion. They tell us how hard and how long they work, about the sacrifices they make, and about the terrible trials and tribulations they endure in the service of the sick and needy. But consumers have come to understand that beneath the white coat, behind the surgical mask, between the two tubes of the stethoscope resides a businessperson. Consumers are asking for the information and tools to deal with these professionals in a businesslike way. In other words, consumers want medical accountability.

That is precisely why we wrote this book. Medicine is a business. While it is a business that deals with illness and the human condition, we must remember that economics is always at play. Every time we use medical services, there is a cost attached. Unless we have insurance, we may not be "accepted" by a hospital or doctor. Doctors have signs in their offices asking people to pay at the time of visit. Hospitals post notices about minimum fees for use of the emergency room. No matter how helpful a medical service may be, the business element is always involved.

For the past several years, there has been a movement among business and government to contain the cost of medical care. The reality is that the cost-containment strategies employed by business and government have been successful in containing costs—but only for some businesses and the federal government. They have had very little effect on the average consumer, employee or Medicare beneficiary. In fact, cost containment has not meant a reduction in fees, but rather a reduction in the amount of money spent by parties trying to contain their costs.

Thirty-two years ago, when the Medicare program was launched, Americans over the age of 65 were spending 15 percent of their incomes for medical services. That predicament was the impetus for passage of the Medicare legislation. Citizens were outraged at these costs, and the Medicare program came into being. By 1996, however, something astounding had occurred. Medicare beneficiaries were now spending upwards of 25 percent of their incomes on medical care over and above what Medicare covered. In other words, the very economic conditions that older people confronted in 1965 and that brought about Medicare were even worse in 1996.

So much for the bad news. Now, what do we do as medical consumers? First, we arm ourselves with information—facts and figures that help us find the best care at the best price. Second, we formulate the questions that will get us the substantive answers we need from our health-care providers.

Here's the good news. In the pages that follow, we have listed and explained hundreds of ways to be a savvy medical consumer. We have given you the facts and information that will help you find the best health care at the lowest price. Some of what you read, you may already know. Other ideas may never have dawned on you.

Every one of these tips to find quality health care and lower your health-care costs works. They have worked for others just like you.

As president of the People's Medical Society, I am convinced that as individuals we can have quality health care and keep our personal expenditures down. As I travel around the country speaking to tens of thousands of people each year, they tell me what they have done to reduce costs for themselves. We have listed those methods in this book.

This book is your key for entering the world of quality health care and reasonable medical costs. We have tried to give you real actions you can take to make sure you receive the best medical care at the best price. (And believe me, I know they work. I have tried many myself.)

The staff of the People's Medical Society and I have reviewed all of these ideas. They are winners. And you too can be a winner over medical incompetence and medical inflation.

Read these ideas carefully. Use them at the next appropriate time. You will be surprised at just how easy it is to take charge of your own medical care. Do not be intimidated by medical professionals when you confront them. Remember that they are in business and so are you. It is your business to get the best care at the lowest cost.

This book will help you do that.

Charles B. Inlander
President
People's Medical Society

Terms printed in boldface can be found in the glossary, beginning on page 121. Only the first mention of the word in the text will be boldfaced.

We have tried to use male and female pronouns in an egalitarian manner throughout this book. Any imbalance in usage has been in the interest of readability.

1

Doctors

Doctors are the so-called gatekeepers of the medical world. Through them, you enter the worlds of the hospital, laboratory and pharmacy. But doctors are also much more. Not only do they determine the quantity of health care you receive and often set the price, but they're also responsible for the quality of care you receive. Even with the advent of **managed care**, doctors control most aspects of the health-care delivery system, including what services you'll receive and where you'll receive them. For these reasons—and more personal ones as well—you'll want to develop a good working relationship with your doctor. Knowing how to interact with a doctor makes you a smarter consumer, improving your prospects of getting high-quality care. By working carefully and assertively with your practitioner, you can increase your chances of receiving high-quality medical care and greatly lower your health costs.

First things first—how do you go about looking for Dr. Right? The fact of the matter is that most consumers spend more time selecting a roofer than they do choosing someone to look after their health. Choosing a doctor isn't easy. It's a process filled with questions, both for the prospective doctor and for yourself, but the savvy consumer will realize that the right choice will save money and perhaps even a life.

Begin your search by getting a few good recommendations from family members, friends and neighbors. Word of mouth is still one of the best methods of finding out which doctors are taking new patients and what others think of those doctors. The old adage "If you want to find a good doctor, ask a nurse" is probably a good one but not always practical. And don't overlook your present doctor, especially if your relationship with this doctor is ending because he is leaving practice or retiring. Ask him for names of other practitioners to consider. Here are some other sources that may help you find a doctor:

▶ *Doctor referral services operated by a local medical society (usually county-based).* Not necessarily our first choice, such services will refer only those doctors who are members of the society.

▶ *Hospital-sponsored physician referral services.* Similar to medical society referral services, in this case a local hospital refers you to a list of physicians who are either on its staff or have privileges at its facility. Neither referral service will comment on the specific ability of referred physicians other than to perhaps mention any **board certifications**.

▶ *Newspaper advertisements of doctors announcing the opening of a new practice.* Be wary, however, and ask yourself why the doctor is advertising. Is it to attract patients because she is just out of medical school? Or is in a highly competitive and glutted market? Or has just moved in from a state where her license was revoked?

▶ *Your company personnel office.* Ask if your company maintains a list of doctors other employees have recommended.

▶ *Your health insurance company.* Check if your insurer has any local doctors to recommend or if it recommends **specialists** for particular conditions.

▶ *Listings in the telephone directory.* Doctors' names are usually arranged according to practice or specialty, but be aware that just because a doctor says she specializes in a certain area of medicine does not mean the doctor actually took any advanced training in it. A doctor can practice in any specialty area she chooses.

▶ *Senior centers.* Some have referral services.

▶ *Your managed-care company.* If you are enrolled in a managed-care program, such as a **health maintenance organization (HMO)**, it will have a list of doctors from which you must choose (see also chapter 6).

Here now are some savvy tips for dealing with doctors.

◆ *Check for board certification.*

Physicians who are board certified have to meet additional training requirements and must pass a rigorous examination administered by a specialty board. Since a large difference in fees between certified and noncertified physicians is unlikely, you may as well go with the doctor who has additional training—*if* he indeed does. Physicians know that consumers have become more savvy about credentials, so they're doing everything they can to make themselves look better. So be alert to physicians who play a little game by putting initials after their names. They're counting on your being impressed when you see the initials "B.E." following their names. Don't be; it only means "board eligible."

Another favorite ploy of some physicians is to list themselves as board certified but fail to tell you in which specialty. You have to make sure that the physician is board certified in his main field of practice. To check the board-certification status of a physician, call the American Board of Medical Specialties. The group's toll-free number is 800-776-CERT. (When you call, have at hand the physician's full name and his city and state.)

◆ *Ask for a get-acquainted visit.*

Before you seek the professional services of a new doctor, we suggest that you contact several physicians to determine if they are accepting new patients. If they are, set up a short get-acquainted visit and offer to pay for the time. (We've seen surveys of physicians showing a range between $30 and $60 for such get-acquainted visits. If a particular doctor wants more, negotiate [tell him the range we quote]. Some physicians may not charge you for the time, but always offer to pay; it's one investment that will return dividends.) The purpose of this visit is to find out if you and the doctor see eye to eye on health issues and if her office services are efficient, and to have any of your questions answered *before* you commit to her services. No matter how thorough your doctor-shopping expedition has been, many problems do not arise until the first face-to-face encounter with the practitioner and the office staff, but with a get-acquainted visit, your chances of things going wrong are lowered.

◆ *Check fees in advance.*

There is a surprising amount of variation in basic fees, and indeed, doctors tend not to publish or post their fees for a variety of reasons. The primary one is that they do not have a set fee for a given procedure. (The skeptic would say that the fees doctors charge have nothing to do with their qualifications—they are more likely to be due to the size of the doctor's mortgage or car payment.)

Each time you visit the doctor, ask what the charges will be for the procedures, tests and treatments the doctor will perform. If the doctor does not know what his fees are, then insist that the person who does know come into the room with you and the doctor. If you are in a managed-care program, such as an HMO, make sure you know if there is a **copayment** required each time you visit the doctor. This is common practice, with copayments ranging from $10 to $20 per visit.

◆ *Negotiate charges and fees.*

Most people never think of negotiating with a doctor. Negotiating is something we do with a car dealer or a flea-market vendor. The savvy consumer, however, never forgets that medicine is a business—in fact, the biggest business in America—and, therefore, normal business practices apply, including negotiation.

Generally, doctors are willing to lower their standard fees for patients with limited incomes or special economic circumstances. Mind you, doctors probably won't readily admit that they negotiate their fees, but in reality, they do. Every time a physician signs an insurance agreement, she is permitting someone else to set the price of service. Businesses have also taken actions that force employees to shop for the best price among physicians. By setting maximum reimbursement levels on insurance plans, businesses are telling employees to find the best value. Physicians are well aware of this practice and, because of increased competition, are more willing to adjust their fees in order to get the business.

Here's the strategy: If the quoted fee seems excessively high or is more than you can pay, tell the doctor. Indicate that you feel this is wrong or that you cannot afford such a cost. Ask if the fee can be lowered in your case or if some other payment scheme can be devised. If you have been using the physician for many years, call upon your loyal patronage. Remember that doctors' services are like airline fares: No two people are necessarily paying the same amount for the same class of service to the same destination. And just like the airlines, a doctor's financial security over the long haul is based on your repeat business.

◆ *Negotiate fees associated with a single problem.*

Have you ever been bugged by the doctor who charges you $50 to treat an ear infection and then charges another

$30 when you come back again two weeks later to check its status? You should be. Negotiate a single fee for the whole problem. Tell your doctor at the first visit that you believe the original fee should cover his second look. Obviously, if there is still a problem, you'll pay for it. But if the problem is gone, and the visit is just a minute or two, ask him to agree to no additional charge. Use this strategy as often as you can. For example, if you receive biweekly allergy shots, negotiate a fee that includes only the shot, not an office visit charge. If you need to have your blood pressure checked weekly, negotiate a low fee, maybe $5 instead of a regular office visit charge.

Even if you're insured, negotiate. The more money you save your insurance company, the less likely it is that your premiums will increase in the future.

◆ *Make it clear to your doctor that all tests must be specifically approved by you before ordering.*

Millions of medical tests are performed annually, and American consumers and insurers spend billions of dollars for them. Yet many millions of these tests aren't necessary, say some experts. And many of the tests aren't very accurate. Others have serious risks and iffy benefits. So you may well wonder, Should I have that test? Does my malady really require two or three tests to determine a **diagnosis**?

The savvy consumer *can* take charge and *can* minimize the risks and costs of unnecessary testing. Here's how:

► Ask why you need the test. Before you agree to any test, ask your doctor what will be done if the test results are abnormal *and* what will be done if the test results are normal.

► Ask how reliable the test is, what the chance is of a false-positive or false-negative result and how risks of either can be minimized. (A false-positive result means that the test shows up positive, or abnormal, but no disease is actually present. A false-negative result means that the test shows up negative, or normal, but you actually have the disease.) Mind you, no test is 100 percent accurate, but you should be told the usefulness and the limits of tests if you are to make an informed decision.

▶ Find out what alternatives you have if you refuse the test.

▶ Ask how much the test will cost. And don't forget to check with your insurance company prior to undergoing an expensive test to see if it will cover the total cost.

◆ *Discuss all options before agreeing to tests.*

Doctors have come to rely on tests to such an extent that they tend to order them routinely, whether or not they're necessary to confirm a diagnosis. Discuss the necessity of each and every recommended test in detail with your doctor. Unnecessary medical testing, done solely as a defensive measure, costs consumers billions of dollars each year. Two Stanford University professors recently estimated the cost of **defensive medicine** at $50 billion per year!

Even in the area of testing, negotiation can play an important role. Let's assume the doctor recommends a particular test. Here's how to negotiate whether it is the most appropriate one for your current situation: Begin by asking, "Why this particular test?" Ask if there is a more comprehensive test that will answer more questions. Ask the doctor to explain the risks associated as well as matters like pain or time involved with the procedure. Of course, ask the price and be prepared to pinpoint whether that price is all-inclusive.

When you get all the information, sit down with the doctor and negotiate what you want. Don't be afraid to ask more questions or make decisions that are not necessarily what the doctor might have originally recommended. Make sure this is a give-and-take situation. Ask the doctor, "If I do X, what are my chances that Y will occur?" In other words, come to an agreement.

◆ *Check if the doctor uses an in-office laboratory.*

In-office labs tend to be less expensive, but just as with any commercial laboratory, the test results are only as good as the people and equipment carrying out the test. Furthermore, regulations and standards governing in-office laboratories vary from state to state, and critics of office-based testing point to problems with accuracy, quality and quality control, lack of adequately trained laboratory staff and staff turnover—and incentive to profit through overtesting. Study after study shows small in-office laboratories tend to have a greater variability in test results than do large, regulated labs. Any one of these problems can take a toll on your health and finances.

So be sure to ask your doctor if her lab is inspected and certified. Find out the qualifications of the people working in the lab. What are their credentials? Is anyone a medical technologist, trained in the proper collection and preparation of specimens and the operation of the equipment? How often is the equipment inspected and calibrated, and when was the last time this was done? Here are four organizations that certify laboratories:

American Society of Clinical Pathologists
2100 W. Harrison St.
Chicago, IL 60612

College of American Pathologists
325 Waukegan Rd.
Northfield, IL 60093

Commission on Office Laboratory Accreditation
8701 Georgia Ave., Suite 610
Silver Spring, MD 20910

National Accrediting Agency for Clinical
Laboratory Sciences
8410 W. Bryn Mawr Ave., Suite 670
Chicago, IL 60631

In 1983, the People's Medical Society created the Code of Practice as a statement we believe each doctor should subscribe to. Ask your doctor to review it and tell you whether he will apply it to your care.

THE PEOPLE'S MEDICAL SOCIETY CODE OF PRACTICE

I will assist you in finding information resources, support groups and health-care providers to help you maintain and improve your health. When you seek my care for specific problems, I will abide by the following Code of Practice:

I. Office Procedures

1. I will post or provide a printed schedule of my fees for office visits, procedures, tests and surgery and provide **itemized bills**.
2. I will provide certain hours each week when I will be available for nonemergency telephone **consultation**.
3. I will schedule appointments to allow the necessary time to see you with minimal waiting. I will promptly report test results to you and return phone calls.
4. I will allow and encourage you to bring a friend or relative into the examining room with you.
5. I will facilitate your getting your medical and hospital records and will provide you with copies of your test results.

II. Choice in Diagnosis and Treatment

1. I will let you know your prognosis, including whether your condition is terminal or will cause disability or pain, and will explain why I believe further diagnostic activity or treatment is necessary.

continued on next page

THE PEOPLE'S MEDICAL SOCIETY CODE OF PRACTICE

continued

2. I will discuss with you diagnostic, treatment and medication options for your particular problem (including the option of no treatment) and describe in understandable terms the risk of each alternative, the chances of success, the possibility of pain, the effect on your functioning, the number of visits each would entail and the cost of each alternative.
3. I will describe my qualifications to perform the proposed diagnostic measures or treatments.
4. I will let you know of organizations, support groups and medical and lay publications that can assist you in understanding, monitoring and treating your problem.
5. I will not proceed until you are satisfied that you understand the benefits and risks of each alternative and I have your agreement on a particular course of action.

◆ *Make it clear to your doctor that all consultations with other physicians must be specifically approved by you before ordering.*

Especially during periods of hospitalization, you may find yourself being billed by specialists for consultations that you may not even have known took place, much less that you approved. Also, check with your insurance company or employee benefits office before agreeing to any consultations; some companies require precertification, which means that the service, the consultation or even the test must be approved in advance. Failure to get prior approval could reduce your benefit and result in a large out-of-pocket expense for you.

◆ *Buy a medical guide to aid you in deciding whether to see a doctor.*

There are several good home medical guides available that offer clear advice and instructions for determining whether a doctor's care is necessary. These are just a few such guides:

The American Medical Association Family Medical Guide 3rd rev. ed. Edited by Jeffrey R. M. Kuntz, M.D., and Asher J. Finkel, M.D. (New York: Random House, 1994).

Doctor in the House: Your Best Guide to Effective Medical Self-Care. John C. Herbert, M.D. (Totowa, NJ: Humana Press, 1994).

Mayo Clinic Family Health Book rev. ed. Edited by David E. Larson, M.D. (New York: William Morrow, 1996).

Self-Care: Your Family Guide to Symptoms and How to Treat Them. Don R. Powell, Ph.D. (Allentown, PA: People's Medical Society, 1996).

Take Care of Yourself: Your Personal Guide to Self-Care and Preventing Illness 5th ed. Donald M. Vickery, M.D., and James F. Fries, M.D. (Reading, MA: Addison-Wesley, 1993).

◆ *Do not use a specialist as a primary-care physician.*

A primary-care physician is one who cares for the whole patient and has not specialized in any one area of the body or condition. Adults have three types of primary-care physicians from which to choose:

▶ ***General practitioners.*** Though dwindling in numbers, there are still some general practitioners in practice today.

▶ ***Family practitioners.*** Doctors who intend to become F.P.'s take additional training beyond medical school—a three-year residency that covers certain aspects of internal medicine, gynecology, minor surgery, obstetrics, pediatrics, orthopedics and preventive medicine—and then must pass a comprehensive examination.

▶ ***Internists.*** Like family practitioners, these doctors complete a three-year residency and must pass a comprehensive examination, but they do not normally take training in pediatrics, orthopedics and obstetrics. Instead, they have more advanced training in diagnosis and management of problems involving areas such as the gastrointestinal system, the heart, the kidney, the liver and the endocrine system.

If you require the care of a specialist for a specific problem (such as a cardiologist for a heart problem), do not ask that person to treat any problems not related to that particular specialty. Not only are a specialist's time and care more expensive, but he may not be the best qualified to deal with problems outside of his specific area of expertise.

◆ *Always go to a nonspecialist first—specialists are rarely necessary.*

As you can see from the previous item, primary-care physicians are able to treat the vast majority of illnesses, and they will readily refer you to a specialist if necessary. But in the meantime, you will have paid less for the care you received. Furthermore, self-referral to a specialist has potential problems. Sure, at some time or another, any of us may need a specialist to help discover the cause of a troublesome problem or to manage an uncommon or complicated disease; however, out of the obvious need for experts in fields of medicine has come an overspecialized, fragmented system of medical care. And out of this has sprung the phenomenon of, for example, the orthopedist who sees "the back problem" and not the person as a whole, the urologist who sees "the bladder infection" and not the person's complete medical condition and so on. Specialization profoundly influences the way medicine is practiced. Too often, patients are referred from doctor to doctor to be reassured that nothing is wrong with the organ system of the doctor's field of interest or specialty.

Self-refer only if you must and if you feel that you, alone or preferably with an **advocate** (a friend or relative) by your side, can maintain control over any decisions regarding tests, procedures and so on. But first determine what type of specialist you need, or even if you need one. Furthermore, if you belong to an HMO or **preferred-provider organization (PPO)** and decide to see a specialist *first*—in short, self-refer, a practice that HMOs and PPOs frown upon—you could be responsible for the entire cost of the visit.

WHAT IS A SPECIALIST?

A specialist is a doctor who concentrates on a specific body system, age group or disorder. After obtaining an M.D. (Doctor of Medicine) or D.O. (Doctor of Osteopathy) degree, a doctor then undergoes two to three years of supervised specialty training (called a **residency**). Many specialists also take one or more years of additional training (called a **fellowship**) in a specific area of their specialty (called a **subspecialty**).

How can you tell if a doctor is a trained specialist? A doctor who has taken extra training in his field often chooses to become board certified. In addition to the extra training, the doctor must pass a rigorous examination administered by a specialty board, a national board of professionals in that specialty field. A doctor who passes the board examination is given the status of *Diplomate.* Plus, most board-certified doctors become members of their medical specialty societies, and any doctor who meets the full requirements for membership is called a *Fellow* of the society and may use the designation. For instance, the title "FACOG" after a doctor's name denotes that she is a Fellow of the American College of Obstetricians and Gynecologists.

◆ *Demand itemized bills.*

Itemized bills are always a good idea because they let you know exactly what you are paying for and help you determine whether you are being billed for a service you did not receive. Sometimes, even an itemized bill doesn't give you enough information to make such determinations. Hospitals and doctors use esoteric codes; if such codes appear on your statement, without explanation, contact the business office and ask for a statement in plain English. If you are still not clear about a charge or have a dispute, ask your doctor to verify that a particular service, test or product was ordered for your care.

◆ *Use ambulatory-care centers (or walk-in/walk-out centers) rather than hospital emergency rooms if your doctor is not available.*

Anytime you feel you need a doctor's care, you should call your doctor first. But if your doctor is not available, an ambulatory-care center (sometimes called urgicenter or emergicenter) is usually less expensive and less time-consuming than a hospital emergency room (ER). Such facilities—either independent clinics or affiliated with hospitals—offer basic medical care on a walk-in basis for 12 or even 24 hours of the day, rather than only during traditional office hours. The mission in most primary/emergency/urgent-care centers is to treat minor injuries or short-term illnesses and provide immediate treatment for routine problems—for example, cuts, sprains, dislocated bones, sore throats and earaches.

◆ *Get a second opinion.*

First isn't always best. It's odd, though, that people are willing, even eager, to ask for seconds on just about everything except medical diagnoses. It is always a good idea, for your health as well as your pocketbook, to get a **second**

opinion on any invasive procedure your doctor recommends, whether diagnostic or surgical. Review the information on benefits in your insurance plan concerning when a second opinion is required and covered. Some companies require a second opinion for all elective procedures; however, if you forgo the second opinion, you may discover that your coverage has been reduced by half. But regardless of who pays, it is always smart to get a second opinion, especially if a trip to the hospital looms in your near future. Studies show that there is often substantial disagreement about diagnoses and treatment options.

◆ *Get more than two opinions when the first two disagree.*

If the second opinion does not agree with the first, it is often a good idea to get a third or even fourth opinion. What you are looking for is a consensus among practitioners, which allows you to make an informed decision about the best course of action. A thorough investigation on your part is the surest way to avoid unnecessary treatment and to save money in the long run.

◆ *Get independent second opinions. Don't rely on a second-opinion referral from your own doctor.*

A lot of second-opinion doctors recommended by first-opinion doctors turn out to be professional ditto marks and not all that valuable in terms of independent judgments. This is true in part because surgeons are the doctors most often asked for second opinions, and they're hardly predisposed to recommend sheathing the knife. It's also true that doctors often refer patients to other doctors for nonmedical reasons, such as the fact that they're golf buddies or "I owe him a favor." You are less likely to get an impartial, objective second opinion from your doctor's friend or close colleague. In addition, chances are that your doctor will call and discuss your case with the person to whom he referred you, and the second opinion will be made before the second doctor has a chance to examine you.

To find your own physician for a second opinion, start by contacting your insurance company and requesting a list of physicians who participate in second-opinion programs. Do the same with your employer's benefits manager and your union, if you're a union member. Check the *Directory of Medical Specialists* in your local library's reference section. Ask friends who might have had similar conditions what doctor they used. The point is, shop around to find the most objective and competent practitioner available.

◆ *Explore non-M.D. providers when possible.*

Basic health care can often be provided competently, safely and less expensively by non-M.D.'s such as **optometrists**, **podiatrists**, **chiropractors**, **audiologists**, **physician assistants**, **nurse-midwives** and **nurse practitioners**. A quick glance through the medical-services section of the *Dictionary of Occupational Titles* will find hundreds of professional occupations concerned with treating and caring for sick and injured people. Some of these practitioners support and complement the services of doctors and dentists, while others practice independently, depending upon the laws of the particular states in which they are licensed.

These so-called limited license providers can save you money if used properly. As a savvy consumer, you should always check their credentials to make certain they are properly licensed or certified—especially if your insurance plan requires that all non-M.D. providers be licensed or certified in accordance with the laws of your state.

Check, too, with your managed-care company to find out what type of practitioners' services are covered. Recently, some HMOs have been covering alternative and complementary therapies on a limited basis. These include naturopaths, homeopaths and others.

◆ *Call ahead to see if the doctor is running on time.*

Just as the savvy traveler calls the airport to see if a flight is on schedule, you can save a lot of time (and money if you must take time off from work) if you call your doctor's office and ask whether appointments are running on schedule. And if you see a doctor regularly, ask the receptionist to call *you* if appointments are running late. This allows you to either adjust your schedule or change the appointment.

◆ *Send the doctor a bill if she keeps you waiting for more than 30 minutes.*

The idea that patients actually bill doctors for waiting time is no longer a novelty. (Not long ago, a savvy Florida man sued his doctor for excessive waiting and won!) Medical practice management experts have taken note of this and are now telling doctors that they had better get used to it. One expert told a doctor to adjust the patient's bill for the next office visit. In short, value your time and remember that if you end up not seeing the doctor, you have lost not only the time in the waiting room, but also the time it took you to get there and back.

◆ *Use a doctor with separate waiting rooms for sick and well visits.*

More and more doctors are offering this convenience, particularly for children. Doctors' offices are prime places to pick up illnesses, and more illnesses mean more money. How smart is it to pay to see a doctor, then pay again for something you "caught" in the waiting room? If your doctor doesn't provide such a service, recommend that he do so.

◆ *Make sure the doctor accepts your insurance coverage.*

Always confirm, at the time you make the appointment, that the doctor accepts the health insurance that you carry *and* will accept your insurance reimbursement as "payment in full," less required copayments or **deductibles**. These three little words can lead to trouble if you and your doctor's billing staff are using the same words but speaking a different language. A simple misunderstanding here can lead to **balance billing**, the practice of billing the patient for the difference between the doctor's usual charge and the amount paid by the insurance company. Clarify these points ahead of time.

◆ *Get a job in a hospital.*

It may sound facetious, but it really can be a money saver. Hospitals often give employees free services—although in recent years, some hospitals have modified their benefits plans to include deductibles.

◆ *Make sure a family member becomes a doctor.*

But don't pay for the relative's education!

◆ *Don't offhandedly substitute an emergency room for your doctor.*

Never go to an ER (except in absolute emergencies) unless you at least try to contact your doctor first. If your doctor does not make provisions for seeing people at relatively short notice during office hours, find another doctor. To avoid out-of-pocket expenses, check your insurance coverage concerning when ER visits are covered and when not. Another reason for avoiding the ER, if possible, is what you may encounter there—less than desirable conditions and possibly a long wait. Some reports indicate that a wait of seven to 10 hours is not that unusual in certain cities and regions; so such a visit not only costs you more money, but it also wastes your valuable time.

If you are enrolled in an HMO, ideally your HMO will want you to use its emergency center or an affiliated hospital's ER for immediate treatment. However, as you know, not every emergency situation is so strategically and conveniently orchestrated. Find out your HMO's rules in the event you seek emergency care during night or weekend hours or when away from home, as well as its rule should your calls to your primary-care physician go unanswered. Be smart and find out *ahead* of the time you *really* need this information.

◆ *Seek telephone advice from your doctor whenever possible.*

Most doctors are happy to answer questions and provide advice over the phone about medication, reactions to treatment or recurring health problems. Ever since the People's Medical Society promoted the use of set-aside telephone hours in our physician Code of Practice (see pages 21 and 22), the concept has been catching on. You can save a considerable amount of money and perhaps unnecessary anguish by avoiding office visits for simple medical advice.

◆ *Get to know your doctor's office staff.*

Many problems can be solved and questions answered by a doctor's office staff, and, frankly, it's just smart to make yourself known to the people who control really important aspects of a medical practice. Patients are generally not charged for brief consultations with the office nurse—by phone or in person.

◆ *Demand that the doctor accept Medicare payments on assignment.*

Most doctors are willing to accept Medicare on **assignment**—which means that you will not be required to pay more than your 20 percent copayment—on a case-by-case basis. If your doctor is hesitant about accepting assignment, remind her that most doctors do accept it and that you would consider switching physicians over the issue. If your doctor refuses, find another doctor.

If you can't find another doctor or don't want to switch, you should know that there is a limit to the amount of balance billing that she may do. This means that **nonparticipating physicians**—physicians that don't accept assignment—may charge you no more than 115 percent of the Medicare-approved amount and not the full difference between their regular fee and the Medicare-approved amount.

◆ *Read about your condition.*

You will be able to make savvy, more informed decisions about your treatment—and avoid possibly unnecessary tests and procedures—if you know a lot about your condition and ask logical and informed questions. Only then will you be able to be a major partner in making your health decisions. And don't neglect to take advantage of a free service right there in your own community: your local public library. If you have not discovered the resources, ingenuity and helpfulness that a reference librarian has to offer, then by all means, do so. Even if you live in a small community with a modest library, one with a limited catalog of medical and health books, there's always interlibrary loan. In addition, hospitals will often let you use their medical libraries.

If you have access to a computer with a modem, get on the information superhighway. Indeed, the Internet is loaded with excellent medical and health sites. And there are many health chat groups on the Internet that allow you to speak to others about your condition. A word of caution, however, about cyberspace health: Be careful of the sources of information. Since the Internet is essentially a large bulletin board without supervision, anybody can put any kind of information on it. That means it is up to you to determine if the information you read is valid, sound and worthy of your consideration.

◆ *Say no if you do not understand, and ask questions until you do.*

Never submit to a test, treatment or procedure that you do not fully understand. You should be able to answer four questions about any treatment your doctor recommends:

1. What is the purpose of this test/procedure/medication?
2. How will it help my condition?
3. Are there less costly, and equally safe, alternatives to what is proposed?
4. What are the possible **side effects**, and what is the probability that one or more will occur?

Don't be intimidated by comments such as "Who's the doctor here?" or "It's to make you better." Every unnecessary test or procedure costs you money, not to mention time and possible discomfort.

◆ *Demand a full justification of any tests or procedures.*

Just as noted above, you can make an informed decision about your doctor's recommendations only if you understand them and you know why a particular treatment is preferable to others.

◆ *Look for free or low-priced community services.*

Many communities offer flu shots, immunizations, simple screening tests, cholesterol screening, occult blood screening and certain other health-related services through the county health department. Also, visit health fairs in your area to learn more about services that are available in your community at no or nominal cost.

◆ *Always ask if it is possible to use previous x-rays rather than take new ones.*

Doctors often order x-rays because they do not know that previous x-rays exist. Keep a complete record of x-rays—what type, when, how many different exposures—and request that x-rays be promptly sent to a new doctor. Even simple x-rays are expensive (and can be dangerous), so they should be taken only if absolutely necessary.

◆ *Avoid mobile x-ray units.*

Mobile x-ray units often use miniature films that require a greater x-ray exposure. Also, these mobile units are used primarily for chest screening for tuberculosis, which is usually unnecessary.

◆ *If you are a woman under 50, consult your physician about the need for routine mammography.*

In light of recent headlines on breast cancer rates, the savvy medical consumer who's a woman undoubtedly is wondering what to do and when. There is great debate among medical experts about when it is useful to begin routine mammography. The benefits of mammography for women between the ages of 50 and 74 seem to be clear. As reported in the January 11, 1995, issue of the *Journal of the American Medical Association,* a meta-analysis of 13 studies that examined mammography screening and breast cancer death rates among women aged 40 to 49 and aged 50 to 74 found the following:

▶ There was a significant reduction in breast cancer deaths in women aged 50 to 74 who underwent regular screening (at 18- to 33-month intervals).

▶ The reduction in the death rates from breast cancer among women aged 50 and older ranged from 20 to 39 percent.

► The studies did not discover a reduction in breast cancer mortality in women younger than 50 who underwent screening mammography for seven to nine years.

Since some women under the age of 50 may be at a higher breast cancer risk than the general population, the American College of Physicians recommends that women between the ages of 40 and 49 discuss their personal situations with their doctors concerning mammography. This recommendation is shared by the American Academy of Family Physicians, the U.S. Preventive Task Force and the National Women's Health Network.

However, the National Cancer Institute, the American Cancer Society, the American College of Gynecologists and Obstetricians, Planned Parenthood Federation of America and 20 other groups support routine screening for all women aged 40 and older.

You should also remember that insurance companies usually will not reimburse for diagnostic tests that aren't medically necessary. This means that any such expense comes out of your pocket. In any case, be sure to discuss mammography thoroughly with your doctor.

◆ *Avoid fluoroscopy if an ordinary x-ray can do the job.*

Fluoroscopy exposes you to much more x-ray radiation and, therefore, should never be used if a simple x-ray will serve. Overkill on tests is a tendency many doctors have— and it's your wallet (and health) that suffers.

◆ *Question routine preemployment x-rays.*

People whose jobs will require them to handle food or work with people are often required to be screened for tuberculosis by state laws. Nowadays, there are perfectly acceptable non-x-ray tests to screen for tuberculosis that do not require radiation, so resist a chest x-ray for this purpose.

◆ *Refuse routine dental x-rays.*

Again, x-ray examinations are expensive and possibly dangerous, so you should never agree to them unless they are necessary to diagnose a problem.

◆ *If you change dentists or go to a dental specialist, take your dental x-rays with you.*

There is no reason to submit to an additional set of x-rays by a new dentist if you have had x-rays done recently. Just take your old ones along with you.

◆ *If you've had three or more normal Pap smears one year apart, ask your doctor if the Pap test may be performed less frequently.*

In 1988, the American Cancer Society adopted this policy, similar to that endorsed by the American College of Obstetricians and Gynecologists, the National Cancer Institute and the American Medical Association. What's a good time interval? A recent study by researchers at the University of Washington in Seattle suggests that going more than two years without a Pap smear increases your risk of developing cervical cancer.

◆ *Have routine screening tests done by non-M.D.'s.*

In many cases, routine screening tests can be done just as accurately by non-M.D.'s—for example, nurse-midwives in the case of Pap smears. It is usually more expensive to take the time of a fully qualified physician to perform simple tests than to use a nurse or other non-M.D.

◆ *Keep your own medical record.*

Although medical information technology is improving and medical record keeping is moving out of the dark ages into computers, it is a savvy medical consumer who keeps her own medical record. In the modern medical age, most people see many doctors over the course of a lifetime. As a result, your complete medical history resides in no one place. There are any number of ways to keep track of your medical record, from a file drawer to books on the subject. We recommend *Your Complete Medical Record* (Allentown, PA: People's Medical Society, 1993).

By knowing when you had a particular illness, what medications you were allergic to or when you were hospitalized (and what happened while you were), you will be able to assist future medical practitioners in serving you.

◆ *Seek out the best medical advice.*

Seek out the best medical advice you can get, especially if your doctor is having trouble making a diagnosis or recommends invasive surgery or an "exotic" or risky treatment. Don't be lulled into thinking your doctor, or even any doctor in your community, knows the right answer.

When in doubt, contact a major medical school or one of America's best teaching hospitals (usually located in major cities). Ask for the chairperson of the department that is associated with your problem. Tell him what the problem is and what has happened so far. Ask if the situation sounds right to him. Also, ask for a recommendation to an expert who might be close to you. You'll be surprised at how easy it is to contact these individuals, and you'll feel much more satisfied knowing you have gone to the best for advice.

◆ *Take a family member or friend into the examining room with you.*

Most of us are nervous, even afraid, when it comes to going to the doctor. This is particularly true if we are sick or worried about what the doctor might find. Therefore, it's good policy to always take a family member or friend into the examining room with you. Why? Well, the most important reason is to have another set of ears. Often in our nervousness, we miss what the doctor is saying. Another set of ears will help to verify what the doctor has said. Also, a family member or friend can ask questions you are too upset to ask.

If your doctor or his nurse gives you a hard time about bringing someone into the room with you, explain that you need the assistance the other person provides. And if your doctor absolutely forbids it, find another doctor.

◆ *Take a tape recorder to your doctor's office.*

When you can't take a family member or friend with you to the doctor, take a tape recorder along. The idea is not to catch your doctor in a lie or to have a record for a malpractice suit, but rather to make sure you heard and understood everything the doctor said. Was that two pills four times a day or four pills two times a day? Having a tape recorder with you allows you to play back what the doctor said at your own leisure, when you're more relaxed and when you can give it your undivided attention.

◆ *Bring a list of questions to ask your doctor.*

Think before you go to the doctor. Make a list of all the questions you want to ask the doctor once you are there. Don't be afraid to pull out the list and fire away once you have his attention. Studies show that the average doctor allows the patient 18 seconds of talking time before he interrupts. If you have a list of questions with you, you won't be easily distracted. If your doctor seems agitated about your questions or the fact that you have a list, explain how important it is that you understand what is going on. Also note that, ultimately, you must make your own medical decisions, and the only way that can be done is with information.

2

Drugs

You don't need to be an economist to know that the cost of prescription drugs has gone through the roof. In the 1980s, the overall inflation rate was 58 percent, while drug prices increased a whopping 152 percent. In the early 1990s, it was a different story, as the inflation rate fell from 7.8 percent to around 3.7 percent by mid-decade. However, this did not necessarily mean consumers were given a price break.

What is a bitter pill for you, the consumer, to swallow is a prescription for profit for the drug manufacturing industry. A 1995 report by Families USA, a Washington-based public interest group, revealed that the profit rate for the manufacturers of the 20 top-selling prescription drugs was five times higher than the median profit rate for all Fortune 500 companies—15 percent versus 3 percent.

How can you stay on the winning side in this multibillion-dollar-a-year industry? Think smart and know where to go to find out whether the drug your doctor prescribes for you is the best, most effective medication for your condition. Granted, in a nation that fills approximately 2.3 billion prescriptions each year and has some 2,500 drugs on the market, even the wisest of medical consumers cannot become familiar with the names of all the available prescription and **over-the-counter (OTC) drugs**. But arm yourself with information on as many "fronts" as you can: everything from choosing the best pharmacist and comparison-shopping for OTC, brand-name and **generic drugs** to avoiding costly and potentially dangerous medication errors.

◆ ***Know your pharmacist.***

A pharmacist can be an invaluable resource for information regarding drugs—any **interactions** to be aware of, alternative forms of the same drug (i.e., liquid or pill) and less expensive alternatives. The pharmacist is the most readily accessible health-care professional most of us have—a highly trained drug expert who probably knows more than your own physician about the relative benefits and risks of various drugs. With the greater complexity of today's medications and, in some cases, the greater potency, the savvy medical consumer will find a competent and communicative pharmacist. It's also smart to talk with your pharmacist, for the better she knows you, the more she will be able to help.

◆ ***Shop around for prescription prices.***

Prescription drug prices vary about as much as a nervous stock market, and it's no secret that most prescription medications go up in cost every year. So now, more than ever, you have got to find better prices for the medications you need. Contact the large chain pharmacies in your area first since they usually offer better discounts because of their bulk-buying practices. Also, consider nontraditional prescription drug outlets such as Wal-Mart or K-Mart. Often, they use their pharmacy departments as loss leaders, selling certain prescriptions below wholesale cost as a way to lure you into the store. And even if you have an insured prescription plan where you work, shopping for the lowest drug price is important, especially if you have a copayment based on a percentage of the total cost.

WHAT A GOOD PHARMACIST DOES: A CHECKLIST

✔ Reads doctors' prescriptions, fills them, labels them and charges appropriately.

✔ Keeps important family medication records, called patient medication profiles, and uses them to prevent allergic reactions to drugs, dangerous interactions, duplicate medications and drug abuse.

✔ Advises, both in person and in writing, how to use prescription and nonprescription medication; how and when to take it; what the possible side effects are; what the shelf life is; how to store the medication; and whether there is potential for dangerous interactions with foods and/or other medications.

✔ Answers your questions about the staggering variety of medicines, remedies, tonics, pills, elixirs, lotions, salves, capsules and powders on the market.

✔ Advises you, when necessary, to seek a medical practitioner's help.

◆ *Buy generic prescription drugs.*

A generic drug (the name of which is usually a condensed version of the drug's original chemical name) is one whose active ingredients duplicate those of the brand-name product. While a generic does not have to be the same size, shape or color of the brand name, by law it does have to be bioequivalent. A generic cannot differ from the pioneer drug by more than 20 percent in either the speed or amount of absorption.

On the average, generic drugs are 30 percent cheaper than their brand-name cousins—even 50 to 70 percent cheaper than the more expensive medicines. Mind you, the generic is *usually* cheaper than the brand-name drug, but always check with your doctor or pharmacist to determine whether a generic form of the drug you need is available, safe and less expensive. Also, since laws vary across the country, ask what your state's law is concerning the substitution of generic for brand-name drugs. For more information about generic drugs in general or specific generic products, talk to your pharmacist.

◆ *Buy store-brand over-the-counter drugs.*

Many pharmacies and some grocery store chains purchase OTC drugs in bulk and package them under their own store's brand name or label. Compare prices of brand-name items with those of the less expensive, but identical, store-brand items.

10 OF THE MOST COMMONLY PRESCRIBED DRUGS AND THEIR GENERIC VERSIONS

Brand Name/Generic Name	*Usage*
Amoxil/amoxicillin	antibiotic
Keflex/cephalexin	antibiotic
Lanoxin/digoxin	heart
Lasix/furosemide	diuretic
Premarin/conjugated estrogen	hormone replacement
Procardia XL/nifedipine	high blood pressure, angina
Synthroid/levothyroxine	thyroid hormone
Trimox/amoxicillin	antibiotic
Tylenol 3/acetaminophen with codeine	pain relief
Xanax/alprazolam	tranquilizer

But before you plunk down your cash for an OTC remedy with possibly questionable effectiveness, find out if a formerly prescription-only drug is available without a prescription. As the Food and Drug Administration (FDA) lifted the prescription-only restriction from many products (most notably **decongestants**, antacids and hydrocortisone), OTC medications became available to treat the same symptoms that prescription drugs treated. The effectiveness of these medications has been proven, and it makes sense to spend your money on these products.

Indeed, Americans treat their ailments without professional help and with nonprescription medicines some 60 percent of the time, according to *American Pharmacy* magazine. Before you self-medicate, however, talk with your doctor or pharmacist about similar OTC drugs. As for the FDA's stamp of approval or its eagerness to remove a suspect drug from the market, let's just say that ineffective and marginally effective drugs do exist.

A word of warning, though: The savvy medical consumer makes a point of consulting a pharmacist or physician before buying any OTC preparations for babies, young children, the elderly, debilitated persons or pregnant or breast-feeding women.

◆ *Buy single-ingredient OTC drugs.*

Many OTC drugs are preparations containing several drugs—for example, a cold medication that combines an **antihistamine** with a decongestant. It is less expensive to purchase a decongestant and an antihistamine separately because often you will need only one of these to treat your symptoms and because mixtures can be more expensive.

Here are a few other wise strategies for selecting the best OTC drugs and getting the most for your money:

▶ Find out the risks or side effects of any OTC drugs you're considering buying and taking.

▶ Ask about potentially dangerous interactions between OTC medications and any prescription drugs you may be taking. Common products such as nose drops, antacids and aspirin can interfere with prescription drugs.

▶ Go over with your pharmacist the label instructions of any medication so that you can be sure you're taking it wisely and appropriately, especially if you're taking drug preparations in forms you do not normally use or fully understand—suppositories or prolonged-release tablets, for instance.

◆ *Break the code.*

What we are talking about is the shorthand code that doctors, pharmacists and nurses share as part of a long tradition of cryptic communication that excludes consumers. Particularly prominent are the medical abbreviations that are scrawled across prescription forms. Here's a list of some Latin directions to pharmacists and abbreviations that turn up frequently on prescription sheets (some doctors may use variations of these symbols):

Abbreviation (on Prescription)	*English Meaning*
ad lib.	as needed
a.c.	before meals
p.c.	after meals
b.i.d.	twice a day
t.i.d.	three times a day
q.i.d.	four times a day
h.s.	at bedtime
p.o.	orally (by mouth)
q.4h	every four hours
q.8h	every eight hours
ut dict.	as directed by doctor
OD	right eye (drops)
OS	left eye (drops)
OU	both eyes (drops)

◆ *Ask for an initial one- to two-day supply of any new prescription to check for side effects.*

Since the possibility exists for an **adverse reaction** to *any* medication, you will save your health and money if you initially request only a one- to two-day supply of a new prescription. You can pick up the remainder of the prescription (and pay for it) the next day if no adverse reaction occurs.

◆ *Ask your doctor for free samples.*

Physicians regularly receive free samples of prescription and OTC medications from pharmaceutical company representatives. Think of it as a test drive, something any savvy consumer would do first.

◆ *Purchase drugs directly from your doctor.*

Let us first say that the practice called physician dispensing is not without its critics; indeed, the entire issue has raised quite a hue and cry in the prescription drug industry—in part because it upsets the so-called natural order of business wherein doctors prescribe and pharmacists dispense. The pharmacists call it an encroachment on their territory and a source of potential harm to consumers. Meanwhile, the doctors call it good for their patients and bottom-line smart for their incomes.

What has made this a growth industry is a relatively new business called **repackaging**: Companies (called repackagers) buy drugs in bulk at wholesale costs from drug manufacturers, then resell to doctors in convenient, safety-sealed containers, ready for on-the-spot dispensing to their patients.

The savvy medical consumer will get all the facts before buying and taking any prescription drug dispensed by her physician:

▶ Compare the doctor's prices with those of area drugstores to determine whether there is an economic advantage.

▶ Verify if anyone in the doctor's office assures that the

drugs dispensed are the right ones, the dosages correct and the directions clear, complete and accurate. (After all, physician dispensing sidesteps the highly trained drug expert, the pharmacist.)

▶ If you have insurance that pays for all or part of your prescription medication, make sure it will pay for medication bought directly from your practitioner.

◆ *Purchase in bulk, when appropriate.*

Although individuals cannot buy drugs directly from wholesalers, bulk purchasing is a way you can purchase your medications in larger quantities. If you're taking a certain medication for an extended period of time, have your physician write the prescription for a six-month or longer supply, as opposed to six refills. Some pharmacists may be wary if you ask for your six refills all at once, and your state's pharmacy laws may prohibit such dispensing. If you have your physician write in the number of pills—such as 200 or 250—then you can discuss bulk purchases with the pharmacist. And don't be afraid to negotiate the price of a bulk purchase. When you buy larger quantities of a medication, it means less time and money spent by the pharmacy filling your prescription. Some of that savings should be passed along directly to you. Negotiation is easier with a small or locally owned pharmacy where the owner/pharmacist can make a price deal with you. Large local or national chains generally do not have anyone in a position to bargain with you at the local store.

◆ *Investigate purchasing by mail order.*

The cost savings of doing such, according to the industry's trade organization, range anywhere from 5 to 40 percent off the prices at your local pharmacy. Most prescription drug insurance programs offered through employers have a mail-order component as part of the service. The American Association of Retired Persons (and other trade and social groups) offers a full-service mail-order pharmacy to members. Other mail-order businesses offer more specialized medications such as **homeopathic remedies** and vitamin and mineral supplements. Before you buy by mail, compare prices with several local pharmacies to be sure you are saving money.

◆ *Ask about any available discount.*

Many, if not most, pharmacies offer senior citizen discounts. Infants' and children's discounts are also available in some pharmacies. Ask the pharmacist for details.

◆ *Purchase or use a prescription plan.*

In recent years, the number of prescription drug insurance plans has grown dramatically. Most large employers now provide them to their employees. Many smaller employers have them as well. And you do not have to be employed to take advantage of these programs. The federal government even approves and regulates such programs for certain types of Medicare supplemental insurance, also called Medigap, policies. Check out these policies with an insurer that sells Medigap insurance in your state.

Generally, prescription drug programs issue you a card. You take your prescription and the card to a pharmacy accepting your drug program and get your prescription filled. You usually must pay a small copayment, usually $5 to $10 per prescription, and the rest is billed to the insurer. If your prescription costs less than the copayment, you pay the lower of the two prices.

Even if you do not have a program like the one above, you may have coverage for prescription medication under your health insurance plan. Most traditional **fee-for-service** and **indemnity insurance plans** that offer major medical coverage provide for some noninpatient medications. Usually, you must first pay an annual out-of-pocket deductible, anywhere from $100 to $500, after which the insurer starts paying up to 80 percent or more of your prescription drug costs.

◆ ***Keep a patient medication profile on yourself (or make sure someone else is doing so).***

No doubt about it—someone should be keeping a medication profile on you and on everyone else in your household. It's a system that monitors all the drugs you are taking, in hopes of avoiding medication errors. Actually, the logical site for the profile is your pharmacy. The American Pharmaceutical Association recommends that a patient medication profile contain the following information:

- ▶ Your name, address and phone number
- ▶ Your birthday, so that the pharmacist can check whether the dosage is age-appropriate
- ▶ Any allergies, reactions or adverse effects you've had
- ▶ A concise health history, including any conditions or diseases that would preclude the use of certain drugs
- ▶ The OTC medicines you take
- ▶ The date and number of each prescription filled for you, the name of the drug, its dosage and strength, quantity, directions for use and price
- ▶ The prescriber and dispenser of every medication you take

◆ ***Properly store drugs.***

Most drug items need to be kept fresh, just as many food products do, with cool, dry conditions best for preserving them. True, some people, especially those who might in an emergency need to get to their medications at a moment's notice, like to keep multiple vials of their prescription drugs stashed away—in the workshop or even in the car. But tossing pills in with the maps and owner's manual is a prescription for trouble—and meltdown. Ask your pharmacist how to store the drugs you are purchasing.

◆ *Guard against overmedication.*

It's a fact that drug overdosing occurs in many hospitals' pediatric wards and nurseries. The dosages—some as much as 10 times greater than prescribed—are the result of misplaced decimal points and sloppy computational skills of nurses and doctors who do not understand the appropriate doses for different age groups. But that's not all. Various reports have pointed out that drug overdosing occurs with the low-weight elderly. Not only are doctors failing to adjust doses for body weight in many cases, but they often also are not taking into account the ages of the patients. The operative physiological fact here is that the older you get, the longer it takes for drugs to clear out of your system, so dosages must be adjusted accordingly.

It just makes sense, doesn't it, that correct dosages vary among people just as their ages and weights vary? If a savvy medical consumer knows this, shouldn't a doctor? Well, the problem, according to one study, is that doctors prescribe "by habit, with little adjustment for individual patients." So the next time your doctor writes a prescription for you, ask her to double-check your weight and age against the recommended standard dosage for that medication. It may mean a double-savvy whammy: You'll save money if the effective drug dose is less, and you'll increase your margin of safety for dose-related side effects.

◆ *Purchase drugs from your HMO pharmacy.*

If you are a member of an HMO, find out if it has an in-house pharmacy. HMO pharmacies often sell drugs to members at wholesale cost or slightly above.

◆ *Consult drug reference books.*

To learn more about the medications that are prescribed for you and your family, consult a drug reference guide. You'll find them in libraries as well as pharmacies. A good guide will list the medication by class—such as an antidiabetic or a calcium channel blocker—by chemical or generic name and by brand name. There should also be a section in which the medication is described and the condition(s) given for which the medication may be prescribed. Additional sections usually discuss how to use the medication, when not to use it in conjunction with other medications and what the side effects and **contraindications** (reasons you shouldn't use the medication) are.

Two good reference guides are the ***Physician's Desk Reference (PDR)*** and *The Complete Drug Reference,* the latter published by Consumer Reports Books. Clearly, the best time to find out that a drug may not be appropriate for you is before you have gone to the expense of having the prescription filled.

◆ *Consult consumer buying guides to drugs.*

Buying guides to drugs, written especially for consumers, are available in most libraries. In addition to giving you information about specific medications, they also point out which drugs are the most effective and which drugs are not effective. Using the most effective drug for a given condition is ultimately cheaper. Here are some guides you may want to look for:

The Complete Drug Reference. (Yonkers, N.Y.: Consumer Reports Books, 1996).

Everything You Need to Know About Drugs. (Springhouse, Pa.: Springhouse Corp., 1996).

The People's Guide to Deadly Drug Interactions. Teresa Graedon, Ph.D., and Joe Graedon. (New York: St. Martin's Press, 1995).

The PDR Family Guide to Prescription Drugs 3d ed. (Montvale, N.J.: Medical Economics Data, 1995).

Worst Pills, Best Pills II. Sidney Wolfe, M.D., et al. (Washington, D.C.: Public Citizen Health Research Group, 1993).

3

Hospitals

Where you get your medical care is as important as who provides it. The setting not only dictates what treatment you get or do not get, but also how much you pay.

You don't have to be a cost accountant to realize that certain health-care settings are more expensive than others, with hospital-based care the steepest. One night in a hospital costs between $380 and $500; an average stay costs a total of $3,080 (March 1994 figures). And that covers only the room and meals; when drugs, medical tests and other charges are factored in, the daily cost climbs sharply to between $880 and $1,500. In terms of national impact, the dollars and cents quickly add up. In 1995, $365 billion was spent for hospital care. That amounts to $1,400 for every man, woman and child in the country.

Dollar figures like these are enough to convince most people to reduce the time spent in the hospital, if not completely eliminate hospitalization in favor of another setting. But if you must go in, pay close attention to procedures and medications ordered by your physician, and make sure you know what has been ordered and that you are fully informed of the whys and wherefores. Further, if you must go in, it stands to reason that a close scrutiny of the entire process, from preadmission talks with your doctor to admission and on to discharge, has the potential to save you money and gets you intimately involved in important decisions about your health and welfare.

Speak up whenever you find something is not what you have been told. Be on the lookout for errors in medications, procedures and the like that can end up costing you extra days in the hospital, as well as extra money from your pocket.

Using even one of the following money-saving hints will save you *at least* the price of this book. And that's just savvy personal finance!

◆ *Don't go unless absolutely necessary.*

An unnecessary stay threatens far more than your wallet, as if money alone weren't enough to make you quibble over the necessity of hospitalization. Hospitals can be hazardous to your health. While in the hospital, not only are you at risk of piling up mounds of charges for procedures and tests, but you are also at risk of acquiring a condition you did not have when you went in. That happens to one out of every five hospital patients, and these conditions not only require additional treatment at additional cost, but they can be deadly as well. One of these so-called iatrogenic (literally, doctor-produced) conditions—**nosocomial infection**—is produced by microorganisms that dwell with relative impunity in hospitals. Most develop at least 72 hours after admission, which means that some may not become manifest until after discharge.

You could describe nosocomial infections as expensive souvenirs of your hospital stay. And close to one out of every 10 patients admitted to a hospital acquires one of these nasty, and often preventable, souvenirs. It is estimated that the recovery time necessary to combat a nosocomial infection is about four extra days of stay. Expensive as they are—experts estimate that they add, at a minimum, $2.5 billion to America's annual medical bill—nosocomial infections can also be deadly

souvenirs: Some tallies of infection-related deaths run as high as 100,000 (other estimates are even higher—300,000 or so) a year. The Centers for Disease Control and Prevention estimates that 80,000 hospital deaths a year are attributable to nosocomial infections.

What does the savvy medical consumer do, however, who needs a particular medical procedure? If you require a surgical procedure, you may be able to avoid the hospital entirely if the surgery can be done on an outpatient basis (see page 56). Ask your physician about this option. Outpatient surgery is usually less expensive than inpatient surgery, and you lessen the risk of picking up a nasty germ while in the hospital. In fact, your insurance plan or your employer may require you to investigate outpatient surgery first.

There's also the matter of copayment, that cost-sharing requirement in many insurance policies in which you assume a portion or percentage of the cost of covered services. If your copayment is 20 percent on inpatient services and only 10 percent on outpatient services—a not unlikely scenario—it's to your advantage to select the outpatient setting.

◆ *Make sure hospital personnel wash their hands before touching you.*

Of all the potentially protective measures you can take (or insist that your caregivers take), this one merits its own individual mention. Why? Well, because most of the hospital-acquired infections are gotten from the contaminated hands of doctors, nurses and other hospital personnel. The Institute for Child Health Policy and others report that many hospital workers who come in direct contact with patients don't take the time, or are not concerned enough, to perform the simplest and best known of precautionary actions. And doctors are among the worst offenders. You can greatly lower your chances of catching such an infection—and paying for its treatment—simply by refusing to allow hospital personnel to care for you until they have washed their hands.

◆ ***Protect yourself from nosocomial infections.***

There is no surefire defense for you if the rest of the hospital is a vast and bubbling breeding ground. So the first step is to try to gain admission to a hospital that has a good (meaning low) nosocomial infection record. Ask your doctor about it. Contact your local department of health. Ask the hospital directly, but be on your guard if the hospital paints too rosy a picture. That may mean that the staff is not properly surveying the facility's infection rate, or not surveying it at all. Ask to speak to the infection officer at the hospital. (If it doesn't have one, don't check in!)

The other line of defense is to be informed. Remember that a savvy medical consumer is armed with information. Know the work areas of the hospital where you are at higher risk:

▶ *Hemodialysis unit.* The equipment here can be a source of hepatitis B, a virulent organism that is difficult to destroy.

▶ *Infant nursery.*

▶ *Intensive care unit.* Usually occupied by patients who are extremely weak and thus susceptible to infection, this unit is operated under emergency measures that often have to forsake pristine sanitary procedures in order to save a life.

▶ *Operating room.*

Nosocomial infections can also pass to patients via the procedural chain of the food services department, due to any one or more factors—nearly all of them with their roots in human error. Studies also point to other work areas in the hospital that, because of persistently poor and unprofessional hygiene practices, are breeding grounds, too: the central service department (the unit responsible for processing, storing and dispensing hospital supplies); the pharmacy; the laundry; and the laboratory (where, more than one story goes, workers have to be admonished not to keep their lunches in the same refrigerators as the ones that contain serum or other specimens).

◆ *Assert yourself.*

While it is true that one-third of all infections treated in hospitals are nosocomial infections, it is also estimated that as many as half are preventable. The savvy medical consumer is, where necessary, assertive. Here are some actions you can take while in the hospital:

▶ If your roommate becomes infected or if you are concerned that what he has could possibly be transmitted to you via the air or through the use of a common bathroom, ask your doctor or the staff nurse-epidemiologist about your risks. Change your room at once if there is any chance you might become infected, because once you are infected, it is too late.

▶ If you are undergoing surgery or a procedure that requires the removal of hair, refuse to be shaven the night before surgery. One study indicates that among people shaved the day prior to their operations, the nosocomial infection rate is 5.6 percent. Chemical depilatories reduce the rate to just 0.6 percent. Using barber clippers to remove hair the morning of surgery yields a low infection rate, too.

▶ Question whether shaving or clipping is necessary at all. Maybe not—and especially when it comes to ob-gyn situations. Removing hair before vaginal delivery or surgery in that area is probably uncalled for, because the old idea that hair creates a climate for infection is unsubstantiated by clinical studies.

▶ Have nurses regularly check the drainage of urinary catheters to help maintain cleanliness.

◆ *If you deliver your baby in the hospital, get her out of there as soon as possible.*

Sure, you've heard that new mothers and their babies are being kicked out of hospitals in less than a day. And you've read that any number of states and the federal government have passed laws assuring mothers-to-be that they will get at least two days in the hospital for uncomplicated childbirth and up to five days for **cesarean section (c-section)** deliveries. But don't fall victim to the hysteria. A woman and her baby should only stay in the hospital as long as is necessary to ensure health. And studies show that amount of time is very short, a day or so in most cases.

Birthing in hospitals exposes infants to the full range of hospital-acquired infections to which adults are exposed. Upper-respiratory and staph infections are common in hospital nurseries. And aside from the worry you will expend, you are required to pay for the necessary care to treat these infections. So the sooner that mother and child leave the hospital, the less chance that either will acquire an unnecessary and expensive infection.

And remember that both doctors and hospitals are legally liable if they force you or your baby to leave before either one of you is medically ready. Remind them of this fact if you feel you're being rushed out the door.

◆ *Refuse admission tests that are not pertinent to your illness or the reason for your hospitalization.*

Most hospitals routinely require a variety of blood and urine tests and an x-ray upon admission, whatever your age and physical health and whether or not you need them. The American College of Radiology has urged that chest x-rays be eliminated as a routine procedure for hospital admissions, tuberculosis screening and preemployment physicals, and as a general rule, it's good to avoid x-rays unless absolutely necessary because of the dangers associated with excessive radiation. It is in the best interest of your physical and financial health to refuse unnecessary routine testing.

◆ *Use outpatient services.*

Many invasive diagnostic tests and simple surgeries can be done on an outpatient basis, an arrangement whereby you arrive in the morning for the procedure and are back home again in the afternoon or evening. As an outpatient, you are not admitted to the hospital, but you receive hospital care (for example, laboratory work and x-rays) without occupying a hospital bed or without receiving room, board or general nursing care. The growth in outpatient care has been so phenomenal that more and more insurance companies are requiring that certain procedures be done on an outpatient basis—mainly because of the cost savings associated with that setting versus inpatient care. Make sure that you know the requirements and limitations of your insurance coverage; otherwise, you may end up paying substantial out-of-pocket costs. Remember that the less time you spend in the hospital, generally the cheaper it will be—and as we discussed before, the less likely you are to acquire a nosocomial infection.

But a word of caution about outpatient procedures: Outpatient facilities come in two forms—hospital owned and operated and privately owned (usually a physician or group of doctors own it). There may be a big difference in quality between the two. Hospital-owned facilities are usually viewed as part of the hospital, whether on the grounds or miles away. As such, when the hospital is inspected for licensure and accreditation, the outpatient program and facilities are also reviewed. Plus, the doctors affiliated with the outpatient program have gone through the hospital's review process, which carefully screens the doctor for competence and training.

This is not necessarily the case with privately owned outpatient facilities. Often, they are owned by a lone doctor who may or may not have an affiliation with a hospital. In addition, states inspect privately owned facilities for health and safety and little else. They tend not to be accredited by any organization. And while most insurance companies will pay your bill at one of these facilities, that in itself is no grounds to be reassured.

So buyer beware! There are many excellent privately owned outpatient facilities, and there are some less-than-wonderful hospital-owned outpatient programs. Look carefully before you say yes and ask a lot of questions.

◆ *Don't stay overnight for diagnostic tests.*

Most diagnostic tests can be done on an outpatient basis, in and out in one day. Again, if you don't have to spend a night in the hospital, don't do it. Remember that any stay in a hospital entails money *and* potential exposure to unwanted illness.

◆ *Go to the hospital that does the largest number of the procedure that you need.*

Studies have shown that you are less likely to suffer complications or die if you have your surgery or other invasive procedure done at a hospital that performs a large number (some experts recommend at least 200 per year) of such procedures. You save yourself a lot of money and untold amounts of suffering if you do what you can to assure the best outcome from the start. After all, you pay the price in more than dollars for their mistakes or inadequacies. To find out how often a particular procedure is done at a hospital, call and ask to speak with the medical director.

◆ *Avoid hospital price gouging.*

As recently as the early 1990s, we would have told you to avoid **for-profit** hospitals. Studies at the time found that they were 23 percent more expensive than their **nonprofit** counterparts. But today, that is not the case. In fact, with most hospitals less than half full (in 1995, only 45 percent of hospital beds were full on any given day), every hospital is in a cost-cutting struggle to stay open. That means you have to be especially careful about hospital price gouging.

It's not unusual to see a $2 pill you get at your local drugstore priced at $29 in the hospital. A toothbrush can cost as much as a defense department wrench. Even if you're fully insured and even if Medicare and Medicaid say they cover it all, the fact is that you will ultimately pay for this gouging in the form of increased premiums or higher copayments and deductibles.

But you can fight back. Make sure you get an itemized bill—one that lists *every single* charge. Review it carefully and challenge anything that doesn't look right. Bring your own medication to the hospital, particularly if you're already taking prescription drugs that will be continued while you are a patient. This will save you oodles of bucks. You may have to sign a release indicating that you brought your own medication and that the hospital is not liable for it. Sign it. You're an adult.

If you really feel that you are being gouged on a particular item or charge, and you are getting nowhere with the hospital people, contact your insurance company's fraud division. Let them know the issue and have them look into it. If you are on Medicare or Medicaid, contact your federal congressional representative. She is your Medicare/Medicaid insurance agent. Have her office look into the problem for you.

◆ *Check room rates in advance.*

Room rates vary from hospital to hospital. Again, the basic charge for a hospital room may range from $380 to $500 a day depending upon the type of hospital and region of the country. The cost of ancillary services (lab, supplies, nursing, etc.) can easily change that to $880 to $1,500 a day. If you have an insurance plan that pays only up to a certain amount, say $350 a day, you have to shop around for an affordable room.

◆ *Refuse to pay a hospital admitting fee or hospital release (or discharge) fee to your doctor.*

These fees, which are commonly charged by doctors for admitting you to and discharging you from the hospital, are unjustifiable on the basis of services rendered to you, the patient. Find out whether your doctor customarily charges such fees and discuss your objections prior to your admission to the hospital.

◆ ***Negotiate a discounted fee with your doctor in exchange for allowing services from a resident.***

If you have no objection to having your surgery or other procedures performed by a resident physician, then make that clear to your doctor. Just remember, that is how residents *learn.* But make sure that you do not pay for more than you get.

◆ ***Avoid c-section deliveries.***

One study has shown that more c-sections are performed at night and on weekends—partly because doctors want to get the delivery over with quickly and, therefore, are less willing to wait through a long labor.

C-section deliveries are major surgery. They are not only much more expensive than vaginal deliveries, but they also expose both mother and baby to additional risks. Further, studies show that only one out of four women who had a previous c-section delivery need have another one for the birth of a subsequent child. The adage "Once a cesarean, always a cesarean" is just not true. Indeed, the American College of Obstetricians and Gynecologists issued strong guidelines some years back stating that repeat cesarean deliveries should no longer be routine.

The best way to avoid a c-section delivery is to be as knowledgeable as you can about the birth process so that you will be better able to ask the right questions and evaluate your doctor's recommendations. Not all c-sections are avoidable, but a good many are—and with information on whys, wherefores and options, you can avoid unnecessary surgery.

◆ *Use a nurse-midwife or family practitioner as your birth attendant and consider alternative birth settings.*

At the outset, let us say that, clearly, where birth attendants and settings are concerned, different strokes for different folks. The savvy—and pregnant—medical consumer realizes that the type of childbirth experience she has depends very much on who she finds to deliver her baby and where she decides to have it.

There are two reasons you save money by choosing a practitioner other than an obstetrician as your birth attendant: Other birth attendants usually charge less in basic delivery fees, and they generally will not recommend a costly c-section or other expensive (and potentially dangerous) high-technology intervention unless it is absolutely necessary. For more information on nurse-midwife services, contact

American College of Nurse-Midwives
818 Connecticut Ave., N.W., Suite 900
Washington, DC 20005
202-728-9860

Developed by **midwives** believing it to be the best alternative to both hospital and home deliveries, the birth center ideally offers a home*like* environment, a relaxed, flexible atmosphere and very little intervention in the birth process. Birth centers are designed to provide maternity care to women judged to be at low risk of obstetric complications, and this approach enjoys a loyal following of doctors, midwives, childbirth educators and consumers who champion the low complication and c-section rates, safety, consumer satisfaction and cost savings that many birth centers offer. A 1994 survey showed that, for a normal birth, birth centers offer a 31 to 46 percent cost savings over hospitals, depending on the length of stay. For more information, contact

National Association of Childbearing Centers
3123 Gottschall Rd.
Perkiomenville, PA 18074
215-234-8068

There is also growing interest in home births, and if your insurance plan will cover such services, it's worthwhile to investigate your options. For more information, contact

National Association of Parents and Professionals
for Safe Alternatives in Childbirth
Route 1, Box 646
Marble Hill, MO 63764
573-238-2010

◆ *Become acquainted with the hospital's birthing policies and routine services before choosing to deliver there.*

From a cost perspective, you should be looking for hospital policies that encourage rooming-in (keeping the baby in the room with you) and early discharge (generally after 24 hours rather than two days [see our earlier discussion on page 55]). Often, hospitals charge for routine birth services—such as enemas, IVs and use of the delivery room—that not every woman receives. Scrutinize the bill and don't pay for any service you didn't receive. (And don't permit your insurance company to, either.) By the way, the average charge for a hospital-based vaginal delivery is $6,430 versus $11,000 for a c-section. Both figures include physician fees.

◆ *Do not routinely circumcise your male babies.*

Circumcision is an operative procedure for which hospitals charge between $124 to $148. It is recognized to be unnecessary for health reasons; consequently, more and more health insurance companies are refusing to pay for this procedure. For more information, contact

National Organization of Circumcision Information Resource Centers
P.O. Box 2512
San Anselmo, CA 94979-2512
415-488-9883
415-488-9660 (fax)

◆ *Demand itemized bills.*

Ongoing studies by national hospital bill auditing firms consistently show that more than 90 percent of all hospital bills contain errors—miscalculations that are seldom in your, the consumer's, favor. In fact, the situation has gotten so out of hand that businesses are now offering bounties to employees who can spot the inaccuracies in their bills. The reward is a split of the money recovered from the hospital.

The problem here is that you can spot these errors only if you receive an itemized bill, which in most cases, will not be given to you unless you ask for it. Scrutinize the bill closely, looking for any supplies, services, procedures or tests that you did not receive.

If your bill is going to be paid by your insurer, be sure to inform your insurer directly and in writing of any inaccuracies in the bill. Everyone saves money by making sure that insurers do not overpay hospitals.

◆ *Keep a diary to compare with the hospital bill.*

Document all medications, tests and procedures and compare your list with the itemized hospital bill. Make sure that individual items match those you actually received and that you are not billed for more items than you received. Again, if you didn't use or undergo it, don't pay for it. You'll find a complete hospital diary in the back of the book *Take This Book to the Hospital With You* (Allentown, PA: People's Medical Society, 1997), along with a hospital evaluation form that should be sent to the People's Medical Society.

HOSPITAL BILLING ERRORS: WHAT TO LOOK FOR

American Claims Evaluation, Inc., a firm in the business of auditing hospital bills, recommends that you ask yourself the following questions to help identify possible errors on a bill. Clearly, these do not cover every possible misbilling, but they are a good start.

1. Was I billed for the right kind of room (semiprivate, private, etc.)?
2. Was I billed for the correct number of days I occupied the hospital room?
3. Was I billed correctly for any time spent in specialized units (intensive care unit, coronary care unit, etc.)?
4. If I left before checkout time, was I billed for an extra day even though I'd already gone?
5. Was I billed only for those x-rays and tests that I actually received?
6. If I had preadmission testing, did the hospital bill me for the standard admission test battery even though I never had it?
7. Was I charged only for supplies, medications, therapy, dressings and injections that I received? Were the quantities correct?
8. Were medications that my doctor prescribed billed over the entire stay even though I took them only once or twice?
9. Were drugs prescribed for me to take home actually received?
10. Was I billed for bedpans, humidifiers, admission kits and thermometers that I never received and/or was not allowed to take home?

◆ *Ask for a daily bill.*

Hospital bills are long and confusing. If you are in a hospital for more than a day, ask to have a copy of the previous day's charges delivered to your room each morning. Like a fine hotel, hospitals keep a running tab of expenditures credited to your account. By asking to see a copy of the daily tab, you'll be better able to question certain charges that look wrong, suspicious or too high.

◆ *Make sure you get what you pay for.*

Many hospitals are teaching hospitals, which means they have a staff of medical interns and residents who work with "attending" physicians (such as your doctor). Unfortunately, this means that although you are paying full fees to your doctor, she may be doing very little of the work. You should specify, in writing, that any surgery or invasive procedure be done by the person you are paying for the service. If you are paying for a fully trained physician, that is who you should get.

◆ *Refuse to be seen by any doctor you don't know.*

If any doctor you do not know enters your hospital room to see you, you can be sure you will receive a bill for his services (often nothing more than a quick glance into your room) unless you immediately make it clear that you do not want those services. Find out who these doctors are and why they are there and make sure you or your insurer does not pay later for the services.

◆ *Have a friend or relative with you to act as advocate.*

In chapter 1, we suggested to always take a friend or relative with you into a doctor's examining room. It's just as important, maybe more important, to always have someone with you at the hospital. As a hospital patient, it is very difficult to be an assertive consumer. Always bring along a friend or family member to act as an advocate, whose most important task will be to make sure you do not agree to anything without fully understanding it. In many cases, these personal advocates may have to stay with you 24 hours a day.

Many hospitals have on staff a so-called patient advocate, who supposedly can help you resolve minor problems. While we can't vouch for the effectiveness of every patient advocate, it's a good idea to at least become acquainted with this person. Let this person know that you're an informed consumer and won't hesitate to call upon him if a situation should arise. And don't forget to bring to the hospital your copy of *Take This Book to the Hospital With You,* the People's Medical Society's guide to surviving your hospital stay.

◆ *Die at home.*

Over 50 percent of medical costs are incurred in the last five days of life. Of course, the decision about where to die is very personal and one that many never get the opportunity to make. But it is a valid consideration—for many reasons, including cost—and should be given serious thought.

◆ *Make a living will.*

A **living will** is a legal document that is used to inform family and medical personnel of your wishes concerning medical care, should you be unable to personally make those wishes known. These documents are most often used to limit the types of medical care you wish to receive if you are known to be in a terminal stage of illness. For instance, a living will may proscribe the use of an artificial life-sustaining treatment, such as an automatic ventilator. By law, every hospital is required to ask you if you have a living will or any other type of directive that can be followed if the issue should arise. The law does not require you to have such directives nor does it mean you must make one up. It merely requires hospitals to ask.

There are many reasons, in addition to the cost considerations, to choose to have a living will. No matter what your reasons, it is a good idea to discuss your living will with both your family and your doctor. And prepare your family to fight for your right to the choices expressed in the living will should you personally be unable to do so.

If you do have a living will, make sure you give a copy to your family doctor and any other physician you regularly use. If you are brought to a hospital unconscious or with no family member present, contact may be made with one of these doctors, who can then pass along your instructions.

To obtain more information on living wills and **durable power of attorney for health care**—another form of **advance directive**—contact:

> Choice in Dying
> 200 Varick St.
> New York, NY 10014
> 800-989-WILL

◆ *Bring your own food.*

Hospital meals are expensive (and, frankly, not always edible), partly because of the costs of hiring clinical dietitians who order menus based upon patients' nutritional needs. But if you are permitted to eat a normal diet, you will not need any special food and can save a lot of money—and keep your taste buds happy in the process—by providing your own food. (Skeptics of hospital food—and there are many, including probably most people who have ever eaten such food—maintain that you won't miss much.) This strategy may also be necessary if you are on a restricted diet, such as vegetarian or kosher. Remember, though, that providing three meals per day is hospital routine. So make it explicit that you do not want the meals and will not pay for them.

◆ *Bring your own drugs.*

As we noted earlier, this is a savvy (and easy) money-saving technique. Bring to the hospital an adequate supply of any medications you take (making sure beforehand, of course, that your doctor is aware of your usual medication regimen and has documented such in your hospital record). Medicate yourself at the appropriate times. It is also a good idea to take along some basic analgesics, such as aspirin or acetaminophen, if you use them. Hospitals charge a lot ($3 for two aspirin tablets, in some cases) for medications.

If you are unable to medicate yourself, ask a family member to help. Have your doctor inform the nurses of such an arrangement.

◆ *Bring your own vitamins to the hospital.*

Hospitals do not ordinarily supply vitamin or mineral supplements—and if they did, you can be sure it would be at an exorbitant price. So if you customarily follow a vitamin and mineral supplementation regimen, bring your vitamins with you. And make sure the doctor marks on your chart that you are to be given your own vitamins or that supplements are to stay in your possession so you can take them yourself.

◆ *Avoid weekend admission.*

Don't allow yourself to be admitted on a nonemergency basis on a Friday afternoon or evening. You will just languish, expensively and in no particular comfort, until Monday. Most of the labs that would be performing your diagnostic workups don't do those things on weekends. Weekend admission equals one or two days extra in the hospital, at your expense. Only basic care is performed on the weekend. Wait until Monday—better yet, Tuesday, some experts say. By Tuesday, the hospital is back in gear after the weekend and the end-of-the-week blahs haven't hit yet.

◆ *Complain if you are being disturbed.*

Hospital personnel are accustomed to dealing with uncomplaining, often drugged, patients. If your room is noisy at night or your sleep is disturbed, complain. A *British Medical Journal* report some years back cited more than 20 studies that responded resoundingly yes to the question "Is sound, prolonged sleep essential for optimal healing?" The savvy medical consumer will make sure that adequate rest periods of uninterrupted sleep are part of the care plan.

◆ *When in doubt, seek out the best hospital for your condition.*

All hospitals are not alike. As we noted earlier in this chapter, finding a hospital that frequently performs the procedure you need is a good way to improve your chances of a successful outcome. But what if there is no hospital (or doctor, for that matter) in your area that has an extensive amount of experience doing the operation or procedure you need? What do you do?

The savvy medical consumer will look nationally for what the medical world calls the centers of excellence for a particular procedure. For example, you probably know that Memorial Sloan Kettering Hospital in New York City is known for cancer treatment. Or that the Mayo Clinic in Rochester, Minnesota, has a worldwide reputation for diagnostics. Just because you do not live where one of these highly regarded institutions is located does not mean you cannot or should not have access to them. In fact, if no one locally is sure of your problem or if no one has a great deal of experience treating it, it's time to look elsewhere.

There are a number of publications, including a book published by *U.S. News and World Report,* that rank the best hospitals in America. While this is highly subjective, it does give you an idea of places to turn to for help. Also, don't be afraid to ask your doctor about a center of excellence outside your local area. You might also contact a medical school in your state, or one of national prominence, and ask for their recommendations of hospitals around the country that specialize in your problem.

◆ *Use a community hospital for your routine procedures.*

Most of us think we need to go to the most renowned hospital for even routine procedures. But the fact is, studies show that community hospitals are usually just as good as, and maybe better than (we'll tell you why in a moment), high-flying, heavily funded teaching hospitals. The reason is simple. Most hospitals today are high-tech institutions. Most can handle just about anything of a common nature that passes their portals. While teaching hospitals are excellent choices if you have a rare or complicated problem, they also tend to have higher infection rates, more medication errors and less personal service. You're more likely to be seen by a student, rather than a doctor, and the sheer volume of business that goes on in these medical behemoths tends to make you feel like a condition rather than a person. Plus, you are bound to pay a lot less in the community hospital.

So don't rush for the biggest and gaudiest when the smaller and simpler may be just your cup of tea.

4

Laboratories

Overtesting, unnecessary testing and errors in test results are problems you need to be on the lookout for. They can do irreparable harm to your pocketbook—*and your health,* if you undergo a dangerous invasive procedure as a result of a faulty test result. A former editor of one of the American Medical Association's journals has estimated that more than half of the tens of millions of medical tests performed annually "do not really contribute to a patient's diagnosis or therapy." And the Centers for Disease Control and Prevention has found that as many as 50 percent of simple blood and urine chemistry tests done in the top 10 percent of the laboratories in the United States are inaccurate. Lab tests can be expected to produce incorrect results a certain percentage of the time, so even the healthiest person will have an abnormal test result from time to time.

There's also the issue of defensive medicine. If the term is new to you, it is doctor-speak meaning, "I gotta do the test because if I don't, the litigious patient might later sue me if something goes wrong." Physicians are subjecting unsuspecting (and usually litigiously low-risk) customers to a battery of worthless pokes and probes that would send Hippocrates, if he were alive today, back to his famed oath ("First, do no harm") to add a new canon that would state, "Second, do no unnecessary test."

What can you do? Ensure that you have tests only when necessary and retest when appropriate. Here's how you do it.

◆ *Avoid hospital laboratories and laboratories and imaging centers owned by doctors.*

Hospital labs are no more reliable than independent laboratories, and they are usually considerably more expensive because the hospital overhead (cost of building, equipment and utilities) is higher.

Also, don't use a laboratory or imaging center that is owned by the physician making the referral. It just stands to reason. No judge should preside over a case in which she has a personal, vested interest. Ethics panels and the public just wouldn't stand for it. No government official should give contracts to friends, or hire relatives or purchase supplies from a company the official owns or has stock in. So why, then, let physicians refer patients to x-ray labs, specialty clinics, private hospitals, kidney dialysis units and physical therapy practices that these same physicians either own or have a financial interest in? Why permit this conflict of interest, ripe for exploitation of the consumer?

In medicine, it's called referral for profit, although more hard-nosed critics have labeled it a kickback scheme. Something else the savvy medical consumer *really* must be aware of: The latest evidence is that doctors who have a financial interest in laboratories order four times the number of diagnostic tests as physicians with no financial investment. And a General Accounting Office study found that physician-owners of Maryland labs or imaging centers ordered, on the average, 14 percent more expensive lab tests and 82 percent more expensive imaging tests than nonowner doctors.

How prevalent are these joint ventures, these investments in health-care facilities by physicians in positions to refer patients for tests or services? An important Florida study, released in August 1991, found that at least 40 percent of the doctors practicing in that state had invested in joint ventures to which they could refer patients. Regulations since then have reduced the overall number, but the consumer should still be on guard against the doctor who is more interested in protecting his investment than in healing the sick.

◆ *Don't let the laboratory run more tests than you need.*

You will notice that lab forms, particularly for blood and urine tests, list a number of different tests on one slip. Make sure that you and your doctor clearly indicate the specific tests that you need. Otherwise, the lab may run all the tests on the lab slip, and you will be charged for them.

Routine presurgical lab tests are another problem area. They account for at least $30 billion a year in business, yet researchers have found that nearly half the time, the tests duplicate those that patients had within the previous year. The findings indicate that normal results taken up to four months prior to surgery can be substituted safely for pre-operative screening tests.

◆ *If your doctor recommends an invasive procedure as the result of a laboratory test, request a retest before agreeing to the procedure.*

Because of the large number of errors made in laboratory tests, it makes sense both financially and for the sake of your health to pay the small fee for another lab test. Erroneous lab results can expose you to expensive, dangerous and potentially life-threatening invasive procedures. If your insurance plan requires approval for any retesting, just remind the powers-that-be that a $25 or even a $200 retest can save thousands in future expenses, not to mention out-of-pocket costs that are your responsibility.

◆ *Investigate the use of home tests rather than laboratory tests.*

Consumers are doing more to keep the doctor away, or at bay, than just eating an apple a day. Sales of do-it-yourself medical tests a few years ago topped the $500-million-a-year mark and climbed to $2.5 billion in 1996. Sold in drugstores, in supermarkets and through catalogs, home tests make it possible for you to take your own blood pressure, check yourself for a urinary tract infection, determine whether you're pregnant, screen yourself for certain cancers, detect the presence of the HIV virus, monitor your blood sugar levels and even predict when you're ovulating. In the early stages of diagnosis, home testing offers a low-cost, convenient alternative to the doctor's office or lab, with results that are quick and private.

But aside from the cost-containment angle, such testing is a good idea because it enables the consumer to involve herself in self-care and in aspects of health care once exclusively the doctor's domain. Do-it-yourself tests, however, are not without potential problems—accuracy, for one, and the situation in which your doctor just repeats the test you took at home. Most experts agree that the objective of home medical tests is for you to *work together* with your health professional to ensure the best health for yourself. Your pharmacist is a good source of information on home medical tests and can tell you what is presently available.

Remember, too, that not all home testing requires a kit. According to the American Cancer Society, every woman over 20 should examine her breasts monthly. Also, the most common type of cancer in humans, skin cancer, is largely curable if caught early, and you don't need a kit to check your skin for moles and suspicious and rapid changes in them.

◆ *Take advantage of free testing programs at community health fairs.*

Usually sponsored by hospitals and featuring lots of give-aways like refrigerator magnets and such, health fairs offer simple screening tests: blood pressure, cholesterol and tuberculosis screening; blood typing; screening for foot deformities and problems; vision testing; and on and on. Since these screenings are usually free, the greatest cost advantage to this method of testing is that you avoid having to pay for a doctor's visit unless one of the test results indicates that you need a doctor's care.

You should know that most health fairs are set up for the purpose of getting the consumer to use (translation: *buy*) the services of the participating providers, be they health-care facilities or physicians. In the words of a top medical marketer, writing in *Medical Economics,* "Doctors looking for an inexpensive way to attract more patients frequently sign up with health fairs...just the kind of low-key marketing that many physicians like best." In other words, keep a cautious attitude and make sure the fair promoters are providing a community service—not just an opportunity for doctors and hospitals to make a quick buck (or several hundred and more) off you.

◆ *Make sure the laboratory is certified.*

As we've noted, not all laboratories are equal in quality. One way to help ensure that your test or specimen is handled and analyzed correctly is to have the test performed at a laboratory certified by one of the agencies listed on page 19.

◆ *Find out when to expect results.*

Whenever a lab test is ordered, ask your doctor when to expect the results. When that day arrives, call the doctor first thing in the morning to remind him you expect a call that day with the outcome. Studies show that many doctors are not good about notifying patients, in a timely fashion, of their test results. In fact, many doctors have lost malpractice cases for not looking at the returned tests (and merely filing them in the patient's record) or not making an adequate effort to contact the patient with the findings. If you haven't heard from the doctor by 4 P.M. on the day results are expected, call again.

5

Insurance

Everyone hopes to stay healthy—but since there's a good chance that you or a member of your family will get sick at some point, it's smart to know how to shop for the best health insurance for your money.

Most people carry health insurance, if they can afford it, or have it provided as a benefit of employment. Lately, though, you've probably noticed that your coverage is not as extensive as it once was and you're paying more out-of-pocket expenses for deductibles and copayments. Some employers who once provided cost-free health insurance now require employees to make premium contributions.

While health insurance premiums have remained steady for the last few years (and in some cases, have even gone down slightly), the cost of health care is still rising and will continue to do so. That means that health insurance rates, whether for an indemnity plan or a managed-care plan, will ultimately go up. In addition, many companies, as a way to control their health-care expenditures for employees, have purchased health insurance plans that pay fewer benefits. This leaves you, the employee, facing larger and larger out-of-pocket expenses. The goal, then, is to maximize your health insurance benefits and reduce your out-of-pocket expenses as much as possible. Here's how.

◆ *Don't duplicate coverage.*

Chances are you will not be permitted to collect full benefits from both policies. The insurance companies invoke a policy they call **coordination of benefits**, which means they compare notes to determine who owes what. They split the bill, or at least the portion that is their responsibility, and you still must pick up any copayment or deductible. In essence, then, the premium for the second policy is down the drain.

◆ *Don't buy disease-specific or accident insurance.*

Disease-specific insurance usually covers one disease—for example, cancer or heart disease—and not only pays limited benefits, but may also duplicate what you already have or are about to purchase. Very limited in coverage (and for this reason, not the best insurance for your money), accident insurance excludes illness but does cover medical expenses resulting from an accident. And most insurers will not allow you to collect from more than one policy for a single injury.

◆ *Shop carefully for long-term-care insurance.*

This insurance is also known as nursing home insurance. The most important point to ask is whether benefits are paid for any level of care: skilled, intermediate or custodial (which usually includes assisted-living arrangements). It's important to make sure the policy you buy pays for all three levels. Up until a few years ago, long-term-care insurance paid benefits *only* for care in a **skilled nursing facility**, but today, policies usually cover the full range of services available. The benefits are paid when such services are deemed medically necessary.

◆ *Buy long-term-care insurance only if you have significant assets to protect.*

Many consumers are buying long-term-care insurance when they do not need it. You should buy a policy only if you have significant financial assets to protect, usually more than $100,000 plus your home. The reason *not to buy* with less than that is that the federal government, through the Medicaid program, pays for nursing home care, regardless of your age, if your assets are below a certain level. And with nursing home care costing anywhere from $30,000 to $80,000 per year, it does not take long for you to "spend down" to Medicaid levels. Thus, unless you have a lot of money to protect, it may be cheaper to pay for a year or so of nursing home care from your own assets and then go on Medicaid than to pay many years of fairly expensive premiums for long-term-care insurance.

So before you buy long-term-care insurance, talk it over with a financial planner or lawyer.

◆ *Take advantage of the free-look period.*

After you have signed an insurance application and paid the premium, your state may permit you to review the policy for a certain number of days—most allow 10 to 15 days—before you decide whether to keep it. If you are not satisfied and decide not to keep the policy, return it to the company within the time allotted and request a full refund of any premium. Call your state insurance department if you have any questions about your policy or about your state's free-look regulation.

◆ *Ask if your employer pays a bounty for erroneous medical bills.*

The first question a savvy medical consumer asks is, "How good are my chances of finding errors?" Companies that audit hospital bills for insurance companies report that over 90 percent of these bills have errors in them: the majority in favor of the hospital! When the *Philadelphia Daily News* took a look at billing—again, hospital bills, in particular—in that city, it found case after case of erroneous charges. In one case, a man had his $25,185 bill for a two-week hospital stay reduced by more than $2,000 after an auditor discovered overcharges.

Many companies will pay a reward, or bounty, to an employee who finds inaccuracies in her hospital bill that result in savings to the company. And as you can imagine, it shouldn't be too difficult to find an error. Your vigilance not only helps reduce your copayment, but your employer also benefits from the overall reduction in health insurance costs.

Don't be surprised if your insurer is not overly enthusiastic when you call to report a hospital's or doctor's overcharge. Insurance companies often find it easier to pay erroneous claims than to go to the trouble of auditing the bill and possibly demanding a refund. But you and everyone else pay for overcharges, so be persistent. Be prepared to fight with your insurer over an error in your bill.

◆ *Get preapproval to make sure services are covered.*

Nowadays, most insurance companies require preapproval for any major or costly procedure your doctor recommends. This applies to both managed-care plans as well as traditional fee-for-service and indemnity-type health insurance plans, which pay a set fee for a particular service. This just means that you (or your doctor) submit a request to your insurance company, who will then either approve or disapprove coverage for the recommended procedure. The process of preapproval becomes even more important when there are penalties attached to bypassing the system. You may opt to have a procedure or treatment done without approval only to learn that your coverage has been reduced by half (or in some cases, totally). Remember that no matter how insistent your doctor is, always check with your insurance carrier prior to any service to make sure the recommended procedure will be covered.

◆ *Pay premiums annually if you can afford to.*

You may be able to receive a discount on your premium if you can pay yearly in one lump sum or even on a semi-annual basis. If you don't have an insurance plan where you work, consider asking your employer to pick up part of your premium. This way, you can make the yearly premium payment and obtain a small benefit from your employment. It also saves your employer the full cost of starting a medical benefits plan.

◆ *Check out HMOs and PPOs—they may be cheaper than health insurance and may offer better benefits.*

HMOs and PPOs are forms of health insurance policies as well as providers. Managed-care plans (see chapter 6 for complete tips on managed care), as they are often called, are sometimes referred to as alternative delivery systems, which simply means alternatives to the traditional fee-for-service system. For the savvy medical consumer, the time to learn the rudiments of managed-care plans is *now*—as the popularity of these plans increases every year and more employers drop traditional insurance entirely and offer managed-care plans or nothing.

Health maintenance organizations come in a variety of forms, but with some elements in common:

▶ HMO members (usually called subscribers) receive comprehensive medical care for a fixed (or prepaid, meaning paid before you receive the services) monthly premium.

▶ The services are provided by an organized group of medical professionals who receive a fixed monthly payment per subscriber, regardless of the services rendered (or not rendered, whatever the case may be).

▶ Subscribers, for the most part, are limited to those physicians, hospitals and other medical providers approved by the HMO.

A preferred-provider organization is a group of physicians and hospitals that contract with insurance companies, unions or employers to provide health care at negotiated fees. In return, the preferred group is guaranteed a volume of patients.

You need to find out when the HMOs in your area have **open enrollment periods** and whether you meet the enrollment criteria. Also, speak to your employer about offering an HMO as an option to traditional health insurance—if your company does not already. If your company offers a PPO, be aware that by joining it, you may be severely limited in the providers you may use.

Consider what it would mean to you to change doctors or use a hospital that is not your favorite, should these be limitations set by the HMO or PPO. In either case, compare rates and coverage. HMOs and PPOs may (or may not) be cheaper.

◆ *Use only providers who accept your insurance plan.*

Some health insurers have arrangements with certain doctors and hospitals—called **participating providers**. Your policy will reimburse at a higher level if you use a participating provider.

◆ *See if you're eligible for group insurance through organizations or associations to which you belong.*

If you are unemployed or otherwise without an employer-subsidized health insurance policy, you may be able to obtain a less expensive group policy through organizations or associations to which you belong—and you may not have to look any farther than your mailbox. Many fraternal, alumni and civic associations have health insurance plans for sale. While many of these offerings are indemnity plans—i.e., they pay a fixed amount per day in the hospital or per service—in a pinch, they can cover at least some of your expenses.

Some states are now offering low-cost insurance for disabled and/or handicapped persons who are unable to obtain private insurance. Contact your state insurance department or department of welfare to see if it is available where you live and if you are eligible.

◆ *Donate blood—join a blood bank.*

By committing yourself to the donation of a specified amount of blood per year, you can receive insurance coverage for blood supplies for yourself and possibly for your family as well.

◆ *Join an ambulance service.*

Just as with a blood bank, private and voluntary ambulance services often offer a specified amount of service for a yearly donation.

◆ *Check all employer-sponsored health insurance plan options carefully.*

A happy scenario is one where your employer, as many larger companies are doing, offers a wide range of policies and options at varying costs. Many workers are offered a cafeteria package of benefits and must choose from an assortment of possibilities. Unfortunately, too many people decide by the toss of a coin—an uninformed and hardly savvy decision-making tactic. To get the best value for your money, carefully compare all the policies with *your needs* in mind. Do not settle for less coverage than you need. Your premium for more coverage may not be much higher.

◆ *Pay premiums on time.*

An insurance company can cancel your policy if you fail to pay the premium or continually pay the premium late. Be sure to keep on top of any necessary employee deductions if yours is an employer-sponsored policy.

◆ *Know what your state insurance department can do for you in the way of consumer protection.*

Your state insurance department plays an important role in regulating insurance companies. Beyond licensing insurance companies and agents, approving policies that are sold and mandating minimum benefits for policies, the department has the power to conduct investigations, take testimony, hold hearings and render verdicts. As such, your state insurance department may also be able to help you if you have a problem with an insurance company or agent. Any formal complaint you file with the department will be investigated and, if possible, resolved.

HOW TO FILE A COMPLAINT WITH YOUR STATE INSURANCE DEPARTMENT

Your complaint should be in writing and contain the following information:

- Your name, address and telephone number
- The name, address and telephone number of your insurance company
- The identification number of your policy
- The type of policy
- The nature of your complaint: the premium, the coverage, a claim or the actions of your agent

Make sure you keep copies of everything you send to the department. You must be willing to follow through on your complaint and appear at any hearings if so directed. If the law and the facts are on your side, the insurance department can usually help resolve the problem.

6

Managed Care

The biggest change in health care in the 1990s is the growth of managed care. From health maintenance organizations to **point-of-service (POS) plans**, managed care has become the dominant form of health insurance in America. At the end of 1996, more than 65 percent of all Americans were enrolled in some form of managed-care program. And even if you continue to be in a traditional indemnity health insurance plan, the chances are it has managed-care elements.

Managed care is not a new concept. Its roots go back more than 50 years, when some large employers wanted to provide high-quality health-care services to their employees but wanted to control the cost and quality of the services. It didn't take off in a big way until medical inflation hit double digits in the 1980s and employers and the federal government were seeing staggering annual increases in their medical costs.

All managed care is not the same. In fact, the quality varies from plan to plan and even within some plans. The savvy medical consumer is the person who knows what to look for when choosing a managed-care plan and how to make the plan work for her once enrolled. Polls show that generally those enrolled in managed-care programs like their plans. The numbers drop some, though, if the consumer is confronted with a serious illness. That is when the real test of a plan's quality and service is seen. But if you do your homework in advance, the chances are that managed care can be a very helpful and healthful way to get your health care.

◆ *Consider managed-care programs.*

Managed care is a form of health insurance. No matter what the managed-care model (see below), the goals of managed care are the same. Managed care is designed to provide only the health care you need, at a price you can afford. Physicians are paid either a salary or a monthly fee no matter how many visits or services you receive. Therefore, the incentive to make more money by providing unnecessary services is removed. At the same time, managed care tends to be more prevention-oriented than the traditional fee-for-service or indemnity insurance models. Simply, managed-care companies make more money if you stay well. Consumers in most managed-care programs give their plans high ratings. Features they particularly like are the level of coverage, the security of knowing what their medical costs will be for the full year and the prevention orientation of the programs.

◆ *Understand the various types of managed care.*

In addition to HMOs, PPOs and POSs, there are also **physician hospital organizations (PHOs)** and **Medicare and Medicaid HMOs**.

HMOs are the oldest and easiest type of managed care to understand. Consumers using an HMO program become members of a particular HMO plan. There are now hundreds of them all across the country. As a member, you or your employer pays the HMO company a monthly premium. For that premium, you receive all the medical care you need. That includes both physician and hospital services. It often includes services not usually covered, or fully covered, by fee-for-service or indemnity insurance plans, such as immunizations, mammograms and well-baby visits. In return for receiving these services, the member agrees to use only those doctors or medical facilities affiliated with or employed by the HMO. If, at any time, you use a doctor or hospital not affiliated with the HMO, you will be responsible for the entire cost of that service yourself.

HMOs can be either nonprofit entities or for-profit companies. They come in two forms, **staff model** and **open panel**. Under the staff model, the HMO actually employs its own physicians, paying each an annual salary and possibly a bonus. In the open panel HMOs, private physicians are contracted by the HMO to provide services to its members. Under this model, each physician receives a monthly reimbursement for every HMO member who selects his practice, whether services are rendered or not. Most HMOs are open panel models.

PPOs are the same as HMOs except that they are owned by the physicians in the program. While they tend to offer the same services as an HMO, PPOs may not have as many doctors or hospitals to choose from. They may also have a limited number of services available outside your local area (a consideration if you travel or have children at school away from home).

POS plans are a cross between an HMO and the fee-for-service or indemnity health insurance plan. In fact, a POS plan is the best of both worlds. In this model, you or your employer pays a monthly premium to a managed-care company. If you use the company's doctors and hospitals, you pay nothing more (other than a possible small copayment per doctor visit). However, if you go outside its network of doctors and hospitals, the insurer will still pay a significant portion of the bill, usually 60 to 70 percent. You must pay the difference. On the other hand, your out-of-pocket costs are capped. Usually, the cap is between $1,000 and $2,500 per year. After you have paid that amount in a given year, the insurer picks up the rest.

PHOs are a recent addition to managed care. Few in number, they are like a PPO except that they are owned by hospitals and the doctors affiliated with them. The advantages are that members tend to receive services at the same facilities and often are provided services not otherwise provided by a PPO or an HMO that covers multiple facilities. The disadvantage is that these arrangements are often very local and narrow in the number of doctors and hospitals participating.

Medicare and Medicaid HMOs are exactly what their names imply: HMOs approved by the federal Health Care Financing Administration for Medicare and Medicaid beneficiaries' participation.

◆ *Review managed-care programs carefully.*

Be careful when selecting a managed-care program. Check out the company that owns the program. Has it been in the managed-care business a long time? Are the rules of the program clear and easily understood? Are you satisfied with the list of doctors and hospitals available? Be sure you know exactly what is covered and what is not. This is particularly important if you or a family member has a chronic condition or is anticipating a particular type of care in the future. Remember that no two managed-care companies or programs are alike.

◆ *Don't join a newly formed managed-care program.*

Wait until the program has been up and running in *your community* for at least four years. Even if the program is part of a large national organization such as Kaiser or Oxford, give the local program time to get established. When a managed-care program is started locally, the owners must recruit doctors and hospitals. Often, they take what they can get or what other managed-care companies have passed over.

So, let the company "mature" in your area before you sign on the dotted line.

◆ *Know the program's policy on emergency care.*

Ideally, the managed-care company will want you to use its emergency center (if it has one) or an affiliated hospital's emergency room. But emergencies don't always happen at locations convenient to these sites. Today, most HMOs and other managed-care programs tell you to go directly to an emergency room. Usually, on the back of your membership card is a toll-free phone number for you or emergency personnel to call once you or your family member is stabilized. But be sure to get, in writing, what you must do to make sure an emergency visit is covered under the program.

◆ *Know your rights when out of town.*

Even though many managed-care companies are owned by major corporations and are national in scope, most programs have different rules in each locality. One reason for this is that managed care, in any form, is regulated by state insurance departments. Since each state has differing laws governing managed-care programs, a Prudential program in Pennsylvania, for example, may have different rules than a Prudential program in Illinois. This becomes important if you travel on business or vacation out of the local area. Be sure you understand what you have to do if you need medical attention while away from home. Ask for it in writing and take a copy with you when you are on your trip. Also, be careful when you travel overseas. In most cases, your insurance or managed-care contract will not pay for care you receive outside the United States. You may need to buy travelers' health insurance before you depart.

◆ *Check out doctors and hospitals.*

When you enter a managed-care program, you basically agree to use its doctors and facilities for a set monthly premium. If you go outside its network of providers, you will either pay a significant portion of the cost or all of it. Therefore, it is essential that you are comfortable with the doctors and facilities in the program.

Check out the following before you make the decision to join:

DOCTORS

▶ Make sure all primary-care doctors and specialists are board certified in their specialties. (See page 15.)

▶ Don't join a managed-care program that has fewer than three doctors in any specialty or fewer than 10 primary-care physicians.

▶ Be sure you can pick any doctor on the list. Sometimes, physicians limit the number of patients they take from any given managed-care program. Check to see if the practice you're interested in using is open to new patients.

▶ Find out what happens when your doctor is unable to see you or is on vacation. Who is the backup practitioner?

HOSPITALS

▶ Be sure all the hospitals in the program are accredited by the Joint Commission on the Accreditation of Healthcare Organizations. (See page 92.)

▶ Check to be sure that at least one of the hospitals has an extensive department in the specialty areas you may use.

▶ Find out if the managed-care company contracts with hospitals with national reputations for certain specialties outside your local area. This is extremely important if you need high-level or cutting-edge technology for less common or more severe conditions.

◆ *Know how to appeal decisions.*

One major complaint about managed-care programs is that doctors and patients often don't have the final decision about treatments. Unlike the traditional fee-for-service insurance plans in which doctors and their patients jointly decide what the course of treatment will be, managed-care plans must approve those decisions. Doing so is the heart of managed care. By reviewing decisions doctors make, managed-care companies are monitoring to be sure they are the best and most appropriate courses of treatment. In most cases, the managed-care companies agree totally with a doctor's decision or recommendation. But there are instances when they do not. In those cases, the managed-care companies deny that service to the patient. However, that is not the end of it.

By law, every licensed managed-care company must have an appeals procedure that patients can use to overturn a negative decision or have it reviewed. The procedure varies from company to company and state to state. So, it is essential that you know and understand how to file such an appeal and what your rights are in the process. Anecdotal reporting suggests that consumers win a large percentage of these appeals.

◆ *Learn how to file a grievance.*

At times, you may be dissatisfied with the way a managed-care company is doing business. For example, you may have been told a certain type of procedure is covered, only to be told later it is not. There are two ways to handle grievances of this nature. One is to find out if your managed-care company has a formal grievance procedure. If it does, use it.

The second option is to file a formal complaint with your state's insurance department. The state insurance department, usually located in your state's capital, licenses every managed-care company. Your insurance department has formal procedures for dealing with complaints and grievances against managed-care entities. Find out your rights under these provisions in your state.

◆ *Watch out for medical malpractice.*

Managed care is merely an insurance program, so it is important to recognize that doctors and hospitals are still individual entities and do make mistakes. While many managed-care companies take great care in selecting doctors and choosing hospitals, they cannot stand over them as care is given. Therefore, it is important that you stay alert to errors or negligence that might be occurring in your treatment. Don't hesitate to inform the managed-care company if you suspect a practitioner or facility is not performing at the highest levels. Also, feel free to file a complaint with the medical or hospital licensing board in your state.

Watch what you sign concerning medical malpractice when you enroll in a managed-care company. Some companies make you agree not to sue the managed-care company if a physician or facility commits malpractice against you. They usually make you agree to an arbitration process. The record to date shows that in some of these arrangements, consumers actually win more malpractice cases than they do in court, but they usually win less money. So before you enroll, be careful to know exactly what your rights to redress are if you suspect medical malpractice has occurred in your course of care.

◆ *Look for an accredited managed-care program.*

With the growth of managed-care programs in the past decade, concern has grown about quality care. In recent years, a number of organizations have entered the business of accrediting managed-care programs. Check to see if the program you are considering is accredited by any of the following organizations:

Accreditation Association for Ambulatory Healthcare
9933 Lawler, Suite 512
Skokie, IL 60077-3702
708-676-9610

Joint Commission on the Accreditation of Healthcare Organizations
One Renaissance Blvd.
Oakbrook Terrace, IL 60181
630-916-5600

National Committee for Quality Assurance
2000 L St., N.W., Suite 500
Washington, DC 20036
202-955-3500

◆ *Look for features that help ensure quality care.*

Make sure the managed-care company has programs that help to ensure quality care. For example, you should be allowed to seek a second opinion on any diagnosis or recommended treatment. This is especially important if surgery or some other **invasive treatment** regimen is suggested. There should also be a provision for you to go outside the company's network of physicians when special expertise is needed and is unavailable within the network. This latter point is tricky, since most managed-care programs try to sell themselves as having everything you need. Usually, they do not, so check out the company's policy about seeking independent second opinions.

Also, find out how often the company reviews the overall records of the hospitals and doctors with whom it contracts. For example, does the managed-care company know each hospital's infection or drug error rate? Does the company know the rates of death and complications, by procedure, of each of the doctors in its employ? Having this kind of information is vital to maintaining and improving quality of care. Ask to see what the managed-care company does to maintain quality.

◆ *Beware of slick-talking salespeople.*

Health care is first and foremost a business. In fact, it is now the largest business in the United States. And managed care is one of the most competitive parts of the health-care business. Today, consumers can choose managed care from a variety of insurance companies. The programs are made available either directly to the consumer or through employers, service or fraternal organizations and unions. No matter where you make the purchase, beware of managed-care-company sales agents. While most are honest, they are, in fact, just that—salespeople. In order to make the sale, managed-care sales agents have been known to exaggerate services, customer satisfaction levels and even levels of coverage. To be safe, *don't believe a word they say,* unless they can back it up in writing. Be especially leery of insurance brokers who contract, for a commission, with managed-care companies and serve as local agents. Many of these brokers represent more than one company, and while a broker may be able to find a managed-care program that's appropriate to your needs, he may also have an inherent conflict of interest because he would rather sell you the program that pays him the highest commission.

◆ *Interview your prospective doctor before enrollment.*

This is not something most managed-care companies encourage or even tolerate, but insist on doing it. Remember that the most important components of any managed-care program are its doctors and hospitals. Before enrolling, review the list of primary-care doctors in the network and tentatively note the practices you might select. Ask to set up an interview appointment with each practice. (See page 16.) If you know you will need a specialist because of an ongoing problem, do the same thing. It is not always easy to drop out of a managed-care program once you have signed a contract, and most employers limit the number of provider changes you can make.

◆ *Look for additional services.*

Many managed-care programs offer services above and beyond their basic coverage. Most have managed prescription drug programs you may purchase. Some provide managed vision care and dental coverage. Some or all of these additional covered services may be included. If not, ask about them. More often than not, these extra coverages are cheaper than what you would purchase outside the managed-care program and can offer substantial savings.

◆ *Make suggestions.*

This may sound strange, but don't hesitate to make recommendations to your managed-care company about service, coverage and practitioners. Remember that whether profit-making or not-for-profit, managed-care companies are big businesses. And businesses are always worried about losing customers, especially managed-care and health-care companies. If bad news is spread about one of these companies, it can go out of business in a flash. This is especially good news for medical consumers because it means that most managed-care companies are responsive to your suggestions. So make them. Tell them how their businesses could be run better. Let them know about staff with bad attitudes, bills that are unreadable, explanations that cannot be translated into any language. The more they hear, the more responsive they will be.

◆ *Don't hesitate to quit.*

If the managed-care program is not working for you, quit it. Of course, make sure you can leave without creating a gap in your medical insurance coverage. If you are employed and your employer allows switching only at a certain time of year, talk to the personnel or benefits director or the company owner. Maybe your problem is one shared by all of the company's employees. A call to the managed-care company from your boss might change it. Short of that, make your case as to why you need to switch before the end of the program year or arrival of the switching period. Also, be careful about expecting to reenroll in a fee-for-service insurance program if you have a preexisting condition. The new insurer may deny or limit your coverage. Check it out before you leave the managed-care program.

◆ *Organize a subscriber group.*

As already noted, most managed-care companies are very sensitive to member complaints or grievances. One way to maximize your power is to create a subscriber group, made up of your coworkers or others who belong to the same managed-care program. Group power is always greater than that of an individual, and it definitely will catch the attention of the managed-care company. Start small and meet once a month. Use your company newsletter to advertise the group's creation. Let the managed-care company know you have organized the group. Ask to have the managed-care company send representatives when you want specific answers to questions. Also, let the group be a way to help educate members. Have the managed-care company send someone to explain how it chooses member doctors or why certain hospitals are in (or out) of the program. Don't be afraid to confront the management with problems or suggestions that come forward in these sessions. Remember that it's your program, and it should be responsive to your needs and those of the other subscribers.

7

Long-Term Care, Nursing Homes and Home Health Care

Since the early 1990s, there has been a revolution in the nursing home industry. For starters, the terminology has changed. Today, most nursing homes are called long-term-care facilities. While most still provide some level of medical/nursing care, there are now many different models from which a consumer can choose. The models vary in the level of care provided. Some provide high-level medical care (skilled nursing facilities); others are little more than congregate living arrangements with minimal medical services available. And because of the aging of the American population, long-term-care facilities are the fastest-growing segment of the entire health-care system.

The term "nursing home" is actually a very general name for several different types of medical/long-term-care facilities. It has the connotation of being a last stop for the elderly, but it can actually be a place for people of all ages to convalesce following an accident or serious illness or a temporary placement for an older person while the family shops around and lines up alternative long-term modes of care. A common classification for nursing homes is the level of care they provide:

▶ *Skilled nursing.* Care is delivered by registered and licensed practical nurses on the orders of an attending physician. The person who requires a **skilled nursing facility** is often bedridden and not able to help himself.

▶ *Intermediate care.* The **intermediate-care facility** provides less intensive care than the skilled facility and usually costs less; the care there stresses rehabilitation therapy to enable the resident to go home or at least regain or retain as many functions of daily living as possible. Care is delivered by registered and licensed practical nurses and an array of therapists.

▶ *Assisted living, sheltered or* ***custodial care.*** This level of care is nonmedical in that residents do not require constant attention from nurses or aides but do need help with such routine activities as getting out of bed, walking, eating and bathing.

At some point over a lifetime, one in every five people can expect to need extended nursing care. To make matters worse, very few *basic* health insurance policies cover nursing home care for more than a few days or weeks. Even Medicare, the federal health insurance plan for senior citizens, does not cover what we think of as long-term care. Medicare covers a limited number of days of skilled nursing facility care only and is primarily intended to permit recovery outside of a hospital. So if you or a member of your family needs such care, you must know how to get quality long-term care without paying more than necessary.

What follow are ways for the savvy medical consumer to get the best value in extended nursing care. Knowing all of your options is the key.

◆ *Use home health care.*

Home health agencies can provide services ranging from help with cooking and cleaning to full nursing care at home. For the elderly person with minor disabilities, a person to cook or clean is often all the support that's needed. A home health agency can help you evaluate the help that you need. But don't purchase any more care than necessary.

Bear in mind that home health care is not just for the elderly on Medicare. Many people under age 65, who are not yet legally disabled—and who, therefore, would not normally qualify for Medicare—but who require rehabilitative or chronic care, are eligible to use home care programs. Home health services offer an opportunity for early discharge from a hospital or a skilled nursing facility, and in fact, such specialized or rehabilitation services often meet a person's long-term needs more efficiently than acute care hospital settings.

If you are eligible for Medicare, know the limits of coverage of home health care. If you are not on Medicare, find out what your insurance plan pays and what eligibility requirements you must meet. Generally, a doctor must arrange for such services as part-time home nursing care, occupational therapy, speech therapy and special meals and other nutritional services to be furnished in your home.

◆ *Check the yellow pages for the visiting nurse association and other agencies that provide home health care.*

The first thing to know is that nursing home placement is not, and should not be, the sole solution to the plight of an older person who is debilitated by ill health and who has increasing difficulty taking care of herself. Nothing mandates nursing home placement if there is someone available to administer the needed care in the home or to coordinate delivery of alternative services. Visiting nurse associations (VNAs) are the oldest home health-care agencies in most communities; however, they aren't the only agencies that provide home health services. Hospitals, nonprofit community organizations and for-profit agencies are also in the home care business. VNAs provide referrals to other community services when appropriate.

Familiarize yourself with the various levels of care available in your community. Full-service agencies, such as the VNA and certified home health agencies, offer everything from skilled nursing care to homemaker services. If you're responsible for the full cost of the services, don't contract for more care than you need. Another important point to consider is whether the agency is certified. This could become rather important if your health insurance plan will cover services only from a certified agency. These groups can provide you with information on certified home care agencies:

Joint Commission on the Accreditation of
Healthcare Organizations
One Renaissance Blvd.
Oakbrook Terrace, IL 60181
630-916-5600

National League for Nursing
350 Hudson St.
New York, NY 10014
212-989-9393

For information on home health services, contact:

Foundation for Hospice and Home Care
519 C St., N.E.
Washington, DC 20002
202-547-6586

◆ *Use adult day care.*

An adult day-care center lets an elderly person enjoy a full range of activities—including arts and crafts, games and just plain old conversation—on a daily basis in a supervised setting. Communities nationwide are establishing such facilities, which provide a degree of supervision and appropriate activities for elderly persons with minor physical disabilities but do not provide nursing care.

It is well established that elderly people remain healthier if they are able to continue to live in their own homes—and it's usually cheaper. Adult day care can often make the difference between being able to remain at home and needing institutionalization.

◆ *If you need nursing home care, purchase the lowest level necessary.*

Of the three levels of nursing home care—skilled, intermediate and assisted living—skilled care is the most expensive because the care is provided by registered and licensed practical nurses on the orders of an attending physician. Remember that skilled care is the only level of care that Medicare will reimburse for, and then only a very limited amount of coverage is provided.

For information on nursing home care, contact

American Association of Homes and Services for the Aging
901 E St., N.W., Suite 500
Washington, DC 20004
202-783-2242

American Health Care Association
1201 L St., N.W.
Washington, DC 20005
202-842-4444

National Consumers League
1701 K St., N.W., Suite 1200
Washington, DC 20006
202-835-3323

QUICK CHECKLIST OF QUESTIONS FOR LONG-TERM-CARE/NURSING HOME ADMINISTRATORS

Even before you spend your time going around to various nursing homes and other long-term-care facilities, touring them and interviewing administrators, you should conduct phone interviews to establish a base of information on which to build. You will want to find out these things:

1. What level of care is offered?
2. Are there restrictions on the types of patients accepted?
3. How many beds (for the type of care you need) does the home provide?
4. Is there a waiting list, and if so, approximately how long is it?
5. What type of license or accreditation does the home have?
6. Does the home accept Medicare and Medicaid?
7. Is there an initial deposit required, and if so, how much is it?
8. What are the monthly room charges?
9. Are additional monthly services provided? What are their charges?

◆ *Use Meals on Wheels and/or other programs that are alternatives to institutionalization.*

An excellent program designed to provide hot, nutritious meals to homebound older people, Meals on Wheels is usually operated by a social service agency or community group. The service delivers one hot meal a day directly to the person's residence, and the price of such a service is nominal, often based on ability to pay.

As with a number of other programs for those people who do not require constant supervision or that much nursing care, Meals on Wheels may actually delay a person's need for a nursing home for many years. The savvy medical consumer will explore the other programs as well: *homemaker services,* for people who require some assistance in the preparation of meals or with housework; *home sharing,* an arrangement in which a resident manager and a few older people share housing and share expenses; *telephone reassurance,* a formal or informal system to take away the risk of total isolation for the elderly person living alone; *shopping services,* which entail having groceries and other needed items delivered; *special transportation services,* consisting of vehicles equipped to handle wheelchairs and other devices for people with limited mobility; and *special health aids or devices,* such as walkers, mechanical feeding devices, geriatric chairs and artificial limbs, which can facilitate personal independence or make it more feasible for a family member to assist. Contact your local, county or state welfare or human services agencies for availability of or more information about these programs.

◆ *Use a hospice.*

Hospices are for people who are terminally ill, and their mission is to promote death with dignity and allow the family close contact with the patient, free from the intrusive high technology of the hospital. Less expensive than a hospital because it does not use life-sustaining technologies, a hospice provides basic medical care, counseling for the patient and family and prescribed pain relievers. Most hospices will care for patients for whom a doctor's prognosis indicates fewer than six months to live. Some hospices come to a person's home and provide services, while others actually operate a facility where the patient resides. For information on hospice care, contact:

Children's Hospice International
2202 Mt. Vernon Ave., Suite 3-C
Alexandria, VA 22301
800-242-4453

Hospice Education Institute
Five Essex Sq., Suite 3-B
Essex, CT 06426-0713
800-331-1620

National Hospice Organization
1901 N. Moore St., Suite 901
Alexandria, VA 22209
800-658-8898

◆ *Investigate assisted living/life-care communities.*

A relatively new concept, these communities provide residential care in an apartment-like setting, along with skilled and intermediate nursing care. As residents require nursing care, they are transferred to the nursing home section of the community and, once they recover, return to their apartments. The life-care community covers all costs of hospitalization, so as you can imagine, the services do not come cheap. This option often requires a substantial, nonrefundable down payment as well as monthly fees. Two good sources of information on life-care communities are the following:

American Association of Homes and Services for the Aging
901 E St., N.W., Suite 500
Washington, DC 20004
202-783-2242

Assisted Living Facilities Association of America
9411 Lee Hwy., Suite J
Fairfax, VA 22031
703-691-8100

◆ *Prepare for the financial costs of nursing care.*

Nursing home care is expensive, costing anywhere from $30,000 to $80,000 per year, depending on the level of care. Many insurance companies are now offering long-term-care insurance—specifically designed to cover nursing home care. If you're going to purchase such a policy, a good rule of thumb is to select a policy that pays at least $80 per day for nursing facility care and $40 a day for home care for four years of coverage. If you can afford it, add a 5 percent compounded inflation coverage rider to the policy. Look for a policy that will keep up with inflation. A present benefit of $60 a day could easily dwindle to a future value of only $20 due to inflation. To obtain a list of insurance companies offering long-term-care policies, contact

> Health Insurance Association of America
> 555 13th St., N.W., Suite 600-E
> Washington, DC 20004
> 202-824-1600

◆ *Find out if you're eligible for Medicaid.*

Medicaid, the government program for the poor, is the largest payer of long-term-care services in the country. The chances are that your friends and neighbors who have been in long-term-care programs for a while are having most of the bill paid by Medicaid! In 1995, Medicaid paid for more than $35 billion in nursing home and other institutional care and more than $12 billion in home and community-based services.

Medicaid is the government health insurance program that will pay for nursing home care when most of a person's assets have been depleted. The program generally pays for all levels of care in certified facilities for an indefinite period of time. It can include care in an assisted living or nursing facility.

Contact your state welfare department, area agency on aging or state department on elderly affairs to find out eligibility requirements in your state. Even if you are not eligible before you enter a nursing home, you will most likely become eligible if you "spend down" your assets in a long-term-care facility.

ARE YOU A CANDIDATE FOR LONG-TERM-CARE INSURANCE?

Not everyone is a candidate for long-term-care insurance. Currently, about half of those age 65 or older are unable to purchase coverage because of either their health or their inability to afford the premiums.

Money magazine suggests buying long-term-care insurance if you (and your spouse) are around age 65, your net worth is greater than $100,000 excluding your home and your annual income is at least $50,000 per year. We would also add that you should be in good health; otherwise, noncoverage for preexisting conditions could mean you never collect benefits.

Individuals with family histories of debilitating diseases such as stroke or Alzheimer's disease may want to consider coverage because the odds of needing nursing facility care are increased.

On the other hand, if you have the discipline to take the money that would be spent on the annual premiums ($1,000 to $3,000 per person per year starting at age 65) and invest it, the cash could give you greater flexibility than the insurance policy in later years in selecting long-term-care options.

◆ *Investigate any facility thoroughly before saying yes.*

Even if a long-term-care facility is licensed and certified, check it out carefully. Inspect it yourself. Look around. Are residents involved in constructive activities, or are they sitting around in wheelchairs staring off into space? Are they restrained in their beds or chairs more as a convenience to staff rather than out of danger of injury? Talk to other people who have family members in the facility. Find out their likes and dislikes about the staff, activities and medical care. Don't be shy about asking questions and sticking your nose into things. Remember that you can't be there every hour of every day looking after your loved one. Make sure you trust those running the place and working in it.

◆ *Make surprise visits to long-term-care facilities.*

The best way to know what goes on in a long-term-care facility is to visit it when you are not expected. Drop by late at night. See what's going on when residents are being awakened in the early morning. Come back an hour after you normally leave. Many nursing facilities operate well when they know an outside eye is on them, such as during normal visiting hours or when the state is coming to inspect. It's the rest of the time that you need to worry about. Don't be afraid to be a pain in the administration's side when it comes to assuring your loved one's care.

8

Medical Equipment

Durable medical equipment such as hospital beds and wheelchairs can be extremely valuable tools in caring for an ill person at home—*and* can save you money in the process. Anything that enables a sick person to remain at home rather than in an institution makes dollars and sense.

Now, the bad news. According to recent government reports, some unethical medical equipment companies have targeted Medicare beneficiaries as easy marks for purchasing medical equipment. The scam usually starts with a letter or telephone call to beneficiaries telling them that they are eligible for a particular piece of medical equipment and that Medicare will pay for it. The problem here is that the equipment may or may not be needed, and if it isn't medically necessary, Medicare will not pay for it. And guess who gets stuck with the bill?

If you know what to do, you can save money on durable medical equipment. Here are our suggestions.

◆ *Borrow medical equipment whenever possible.*

Most home health aids can be borrowed from various community organizations. Ask your local home health organization or visiting nurse association. If no such services are available in your area, you may be able to rent the required equipment from a local pharmacy. But before renting, check to see if your insurance policy will cover its purchase. Also, shop around; rental prices for equipment vary from dealer to dealer. If you need the equipment for a long period of time, you will probably have to purchase it.

◆ *Save by owning medical self-care equipment.*

Simple items of self-care equipment such as thermometers, blood pressure cuffs, stethoscopes and otoscopes are helpful devices, especially when it comes to making informed choices concerning your need for a doctor's help. Many are available from discount mail-order companies. Check out a number of suppliers to find a high-quality item at a reasonable price.

◆ *Check out the equipment's reliability before purchasing.*

Every piece of equipment should come with literature that describes its reliability within a certain range. For instance, thermometers may be reliable within a range of one degree Fahrenheit. Some equipment will be more reliable than others. The equipment's accompanying literature should also describe the period of time the equipment can be expected to maintain this degree of reliability without servicing.

Also, before purchasing a piece of durable medical equipment, find out about the warranty. Check, too, if the manufacturer or dealer offers extended warranty protection on particularly expensive items.

◆ *Find out where servicing is available.*

Equipment such as blood pressure cuffs must be periodically serviced to maintain reliability. Make sure that you know how, where and how often a piece of equipment must be serviced before you purchase it. In fact, it makes sense to purchase only equipment with a written warranty. Further, you will save money if the equipment you buy can be serviced locally.

◆ *Check out the supplier with the Better Business Bureau and with Medicare if the equipment is for a Medicare beneficiary.*

For many health items such as hearing aids, it is wise to see if your local Better Business Bureau has any complaints on file against the supplier from whom you are thinking of purchasing. If the equipment is prescribed for a Medicare beneficiary, determine if the supplier is a certified Medicare supplier. What this means is that the supplier will accept the Medicare-approved amount as payment in full and will bill the beneficiary only for the 20 percent copayment.

◆ *Check for sales.*

With health and medical equipment, just as with most other consumer items, suppliers often offer sales. Purchasing items on sale is always a good way to save money.

◆ *Return any medical equipment that arrives unsolicited.*

Some doctors and medical suppliers target Medicare beneficiaries with offers of so-called free equipment paid for by Medicare. In addition, some equipment manufacturers use well-known personalities to hawk various products ranging from special beds to power-assisted chairs. Be aware that Medicare will pay only for durable medical equipment that's prescribed by your doctor, as long as it is medically necessary. The words "medically necessary" are the key here. Unless your doctor specifically orders equipment, do not respond to any mail-order or telephone marketing schemes.

9

Prevention

Taking preventive measures has the potential to save you more money on health costs than anything else you do. Even more important, prevention is health promotion, something every savvy medical consumer should be doing more of. But the bad news is that while 58 cents out of every health-care dollar goes to doctors and hospitals, only two cents goes to health promotion activities. That's all we spend to keep ourselves healthy.

However, you have many opportunities in daily living to get your two cents' worth by doing things that will improve your health. And remember that the sooner you start, the healthier you will be.

◆ *Learn stress-reduction techniques.*

There are techniques—some simple, others requiring professional help—that can help you lower your stress level. Strong evidence exists that those under stress, or those who cope poorly with stress, are less healthy than others. And at the very least, that adds up to a lot of extra dollars spent on medical care.

◆ *Quit smoking.*

Smoking increases a person's risk for a number of major diseases: heart disease, stroke and cancer. But beyond that, smokers are just generally more prone to illness—and, therefore, lose more work time due to illness—than nonsmokers. If you are a smoker, consider also the increased risk at which you put your friends and family as they breathe in your exhaled smoke. Save money and your health by throwing away your cigarettes. And don't think that cigar or pipe smoking is healthier. The increased risk of lip, mouth and tongue cancer is equal to cigarette risk, even if you do not inhale.

◆ *Don't do anything to excess.*

Old wisdom, but true today. Excessive eating, drinking, smoking and even exercise can be harmful and expensive.

◆ *Make your home injury proof.*

Inspect your home for safety. Check electrical cords, the condition of carpeting, the placement of furniture and so on. Additions such as nonslip strips on bathtubs are inexpensive ways to ensure your safety and prevent the need for costly medical care.

◆ *Maintain a desirable weight.*

This does not necessarily mean that you should weigh what those famous charts say you should weigh, but you will be healthier if you weigh what feels good for you. And you'll save money on health care as well. Overweight people not only are more prone to conditions such as diabetes and heart disease, but they are also more likely to need hip, knee and other joint replacements in later years.

◆ *Wear seat belts.*

Some cars employ a passive restraint system that automatically fastens your seat belt; however, you may still need to manually fasten the lap belt. Whatever the case, you're always safer when you properly use the safety equipment that is included with your car. Forty-five thousand deaths a year, untold pain and suffering and loss of income should be enough to convince anyone to use seat belts.

◆ ***Buy vehicles with air bags.***

Despite what you may have read about air bags, children and small adults, the overall record of air bags is excellent compared with seat belts alone. Thousands of lives that would otherwise have been lost have been saved (most without injury) by air bag deployment. As for children, they should always be restrained in the backseat, never the front. And be sure to always use your seat belt in conjunction with an air bag.

◆ ***Always properly restrain children in cars.***

Remember: *You* are responsible for the safety of your children. It's a good idea to take along a car seat on airplanes and other forms of transportation. Injury prevention saves money and incalculable suffering. When using these restraints, follow the printed instructions that come with the product. Not doing so will reduce the safety effectiveness of the product and could cause serious injury to your child.

◆ ***Drive slower.***

Drivers who speed have more accidents than those who stay within the speed limits. Plus, don't be lured into thinking that the recent increase in speed limits in certain states is a license to jam down on the accelerator. Even those increased limits may be too fast for conditions. Be a little late, but arrive in one piece.

◆ ***Avoid processed foods.***

Processed foods usually contain more fat, more salt and less fiber than unprocessed foods. They also contain preservatives and other chemicals. The healthier you are, the more money you will save on costly medical care—so pass the bran.

◆ *Have microwave emissions checked.*

Call the authorized repair service recommended in the literature accompanying your microwave. (Indeed, your manual should include a maintenance schedule.) A repair service should be able to do a quick, low-cost emission check. Microwave emissions are potentially harmful, so a few dollars for a check can save you medical costs in the future.

◆ *Purchase basic medical tools for self-diagnosis.*

You can save yourself time and expense by having basic medical tools such as a blood pressure cuff (sphygmomanometer), an otoscope (for looking in the ears) and a stethoscope. Used in combination with a good medical guide, these tools can help you avoid many unnecessary visits to the doctor.

◆ *Join the People's Medical Society.*

The People's Medical Society *Newsletter* and our many other publications offer you an easy-to-read supply of medical information that you can use to make informed decisions about your health care.

◆ *Plan a fire escape route and hold home fire drills.*

Simple fire safety measures such as smoke alarms—an ample number placed strategically in your home—and fire drills can prevent serious injury or worse in the event of a home fire.

◆ *Exercise regularly.*

Regular exercise protects against heart disease, osteoporosis and a variety of other common illnesses. It will also help you maintain a desirable weight and reduce stress. Joining a health club is cheaper than health care for a chronic illness such as heart disease.

◆ *Make friends and purchase a pet.*

Studies have shown that people who are socially active are healthier than those who are loners. Check your local newspaper for singles activities at churches, social organizations, Parents Without Partners, exercise clubs and so on. Place an ad in the personals section of newspapers and magazines or be daring and answer one!

Pets make great companions, and there are many dogs and cats at your local animal shelter just waiting for adoption. You'll have a lifelong friend and the satisfaction that comes with helping a less fortunate creature. How you feel mentally has long been known to be connected to how you feel physically, and being socially active and having a pet are two ways to improve your health. And remember that the cost for dog and cat food is considerably less than the cost of multiple doctor visits and prescription medications.

◆ *Wear a lead apron for dental x-rays.*

You should always shield the parts of your body not being x-rayed. Excessive radiation is a definite health hazard—and why invite trouble (and additional costs) when there's a simple remedy?

◆ *Keep current with immunizations.*

Adults need to be reimmunized periodically for tetanus and, in some areas of the country, other diseases as well. These immunizations often are given free or at a very low cost through community groups. Elderly adults and people with chronic conditions should consider immunization against influenza and pneumonia.

◆ *Avoid too much exposure to the sun.*

Dermatologists have definitely identified a link between exposure to the sun and skin cancer; however, you don't have to live in a cave. Use commonsense approaches to the sun: Always use a sunscreen with a sun protection factor (SPF) of 15 or more; keep your exposure to a minimum; don't get all your sun at once; and wear protective clothing such as a hat or long-sleeved shirt when in the sun.

For more information on how to enjoy the sun and avoid the hazards, contact

Skin Cancer Foundation
245 Fifth Ave., Suite 1403
New York, NY 10016
212-725-5176

◆ *Wash your hands.*

Frequent hand washing will lower your chances of catching colds, flu and other contagious diseases.

◆ *Take a vacation.*

Everyone needs and benefits from periodic breaks in the daily routine. Listen to yourself—don't get too burned out before you give yourself a break. Hotels are cheaper than hospitals.

◆ *Get enough sleep.*

Many conditions are related to or exacerbated by lack of sleep. Most people need seven to eight hours of sleep per day. Listen to yourself and make sure you get what you need.

◆ *Eat lots of fiber.*

Increasing the amount of fiber in your diet is the easiest way to lower your risk of colon cancer and heart attack. It will also help to lower cholesterol and prevent constipation.

Laxatives are much more expensive than an extra slice of whole-wheat bread.

◆ *Drink cranberry juice.*

Cranberry juice can be protective against bladder infections. But be careful to avoid the juices with a lot of added sugar and corn syrups. Cranberry juice is cheaper than antibiotics—and a lot more fun to ingest.

◆ *Brush your teeth and floss daily.*

Good oral hygiene is essential to good general health, so don't forget to brush and floss your teeth on a daily basis. Failure to develop and practice good oral health habits can be counterproductive to all your efforts at staying healthy. In addition, one unforeseen dental bill can wipe out any savings you've accumulated by practicing good general health.

Buy a plaque removal system for you and your family. Gum disease is one of the leading causes of tooth loss, and the cost to replace lost teeth can be quite high.

◆ *Contact a self-help support group.*

For many illnesses, a self-help support group can be as helpful as your doctor in speeding your recovery. Self-help support groups are in the business of empowerment, giving consumers the information and strategies they need to successfully deal with their conditions. In addition, in such groups, you meet people who share your condition and with whom you can share a common bond. For more information on self-help groups, contact

> American Self-Help Clearinghouse
> Northwest Covenant Medical Center
> 25 Pocono Rd.
> Denville, NJ 07834
> 201-625-7101
> 201-625-9053 (TDD)

National Self-Help Clearinghouse
City University of New York
Graduate Center, Room 620
25 W. 43rd St.
New York, NY 10036
212-354-8525

◆ *Practice safe sex.*

Unfortunately and undeniably, sexually transmitted diseases—gonorrhea, herpes, syphilis and human immunodeficiency virus (HIV, the virus that can cause AIDS), just to name a few—are a nasty fact of life. Most at risk are those people who have had many sexual partners. The risks, however, are minimized if a condom is always and correctly used during intercourse.

◆ *Know the number for your local poison control center.*

Calling for help immediately if you suspect someone in your family has ingested a poisonous substance can make the difference between a minor digestive disturbance and a week in the hospital's intensive care unit. Prompt action saves lives and money.

◆ *Wear appropriate protective clothing and equipment when playing sports or engaging in recreational activities.*

Whether the activity is bicycling or football, protective clothing can spare participants from easily preventable injuries. Preventing injuries or lessening their severity saves money.

GLOSSARY 1
Medical Terms

Advance directive: A written document stating how a person wants medical decisions made for him if he is unable to make those decisions himself. The two most common advance directives are living wills and durable powers of attorney for health care.

Adverse reaction: A reaction that harms a person in some way.

Advocate: A person who represents another's interests.

Antihistamine: A medication used to treat allergy and cold symptoms such as itchy eyes and a runny nose.

Assignment: A process by which a doctor or hospital agrees to file an insurance claim in exchange for direct payment from the insurer. Under the Medicare system, the physician or hospital must also agree to accept that direct payment, plus any required patient copayments, as payment in full.

Audiologist: A health-care practitioner (non-M.D., non-D.O.) who specializes in treating hearing problems.

Balance billing: The practice of billing the patient for the difference between the doctor's usual charge and the amount paid by the insurance company.

Board certification (board certified): The status conferred upon a physician who has passed an examination given by a medical specialty board recognized by the American Board of Medical Specialists. Board certification is offered in 29 recognized specialties, such as pediatrics, obstetrics and gynecology and internal medicine.

Cesarean section (c-section): A method of delivering a baby by abdominal surgery.

Chiropractor: A health-care practitioner (D.C.; non-M.D., non-D.O.) who focuses on improving nerve function through manipulation and adjustment of body parts, particularly the spine.

Consultation: A discussion between physicians about a medical case or its treatment, for which the patient is billed.

Contraindication: Something that makes the use of a particular medication or treatment inadvisable.

Coordination of benefits: A review of benefit coverage done when two or more insurance plans cover the same procedure. The companies compare notes to determine who owes what. They split the bill, or at least the portion that is their responsibility, and the consumer must still pick up any copayment or deductible.

Copayment: A payment required of the patient in addition to the payment made by the insurance company. A copayment may be in the form of a deductible or a percentage payment (for instance, the insurance company pays 80 percent and the patient pays 20 percent).

Custodial care: The provision of room, board and personal services, generally on a long-term basis, without additional medical services.

Decongestant: A medication that acts to clear congestion. It helps such symptoms as stuffy nose or chest congestion.

Deductible: The amount a patient is required to pay before her insurance company begins to make payments.

Defensive medicine: The practicing of medicine with the goal of avoiding medical malpractice lawsuits, generally involving the ordering of many and perhaps unnecessary tests and procedures.

Diagnosis: The identification of a patient's illness through consideration of the signs and symptoms.

Durable power of attorney for health care: A form of medical advance directive that empowers a person to make health-care decisions for another should that person become unable to do so herself.

Family practitioner: A medical practitioner (M.D., D.O.) who specializes in treating the whole family, from uncomplicated births to care of the elderly.

Fee-for-service insurance plan: An insurance plan that reimburses the medical practitioner for services provided, in an amount that may or may not equal the charge of the procedure but which the practitioner agrees to accept as payment in full. The payment is generally sent directly to the practitioner.

Fellowship: A grant given to a medical practitioner that permits him to study a certain area of medicine, usually in conjunction with some specialty such as oncology or surgery. It may be used to develop direct patient-care modalities or for pure medical or biological research.

For-profit: A business that operates to make more money than it requires to continue operating.

General practitioner: A physician (M.D., D.O.) who can provide routine care for a wide range of medical problems.

Generic drug: A drug that is a copy of a brand-name drug. Its active ingredients must duplicate those of the brand-name drug.

Health maintenance organization (HMO): A form of managed care in which each consumer member pays a monthly premium in return for all necessary medical care. Members are covered only if they use doctors and medical facilities affiliated with the HMO and are subject to other restrictions as determined by their agreement. Costs incurred outside the network are usually not covered.

Homeopathic remedy: A medication used in homeopathy, which is a system of nontraditional medicine that is based upon the law of similars and the law of infinitesimals. The law of similars states that substances that provoke certain reactions in healthy people can be used to mitigate similar responses in people who are symptomatic. The law of infinitesimals states that the more vigorously a substance is diluted, the more potent it becomes.

Hospice: An organization that provides specialized care for dying patients either in their homes or at a special facility.

Indemnity insurance plan: An insurance plan that pays a set amount of reimbursement regardless of the fee charged by the practitioner. The insured is then responsible for payment of any excess charges. The payment is generally sent directly to the insured.

Interaction: The action of one drug upon the effectiveness or toxicity of another (or others).

Intermediate-care facility: A facility that provides less intensive care than a skilled nursing facility. Patients are generally more mobile, and rehabilitation therapies are stressed.

Internist: A physician (M.D., D.O.) who completes a three-year residency and passes a comprehensive examination but does not normally take training in pediatrics, orthopedics or child delivery. Instead, an internist has more advanced training in diagnosis and management of problems involving areas such as the gastrointestinal system, the heart, the kidney, the liver and the endocrine system.

Invasive treatment: A medical treatment that involves the invasion of the body with a drug or an instrument.

Itemized bill: A bill that lists each item and service and its corresponding charge.

Living will: A document that indicates a person's treatment wishes in the event that he is unable to verbally communicate those wishes. A living will is usually used as written authorization for the nonuse or removal of life-sustaining treatments.

Managed care: A form of health insurance that focuses on prevention, cost containment and the provision of high-quality health care to consumers through a defined network of practitioners and facilities.

Medicare and Medicaid HMOs: HMOs approved by the federal Health Care Financing Administration for Medicare and Medicaid beneficiaries' participation.

Midwife: See **Nurse-midwife**.

Nonparticipating physician: A physician that does not accept assignment. These physicians will bill for the cost of their services over the amount paid by insurance.

Nonprofit: An organization that functions by earning just enough money to continue operating.

Nosocomial infection: An infection acquired in the hospital.

Nurse practitioner: A nurse who has received specialized training that enables her to provide basic diagnostic medical care to patients.

Nurse-midwife: A medical practitioner who specializes in caring for women and delivering babies.

Open enrollment period: A period of time, defined by an insurer or health plan, during which anyone may apply for coverage and be accepted without evidence of insurability or waiting periods. The period may last from 30 to 90 days.

Open panel: A type of HMO in which private physicians are contracted by the HMO to provide services to its members. Under this model, the physician receives a monthly reimbursement for every HMO member who selects her practice, whether services are rendered or not. Most HMOs are open panel models.

Optometrist: A medical practitioner (O.D.) who specializes in examining eyes and who is able to prescribe corrective lenses but not perform surgery or invasive treatments.

Over-the-counter (OTC) drug: A drug that is available without a doctor's prescription.

Participating provider: A medical provider who has a contract with an insurer or health plan to provide services to covered persons and agrees to accept the reimbursement schedule of the plan as payment in full. The provider may be a physician, hospital, laboratory, outpatient facility or pharmacy.

Physician hospital organization (PHO): A managed-care plan owned by a hospital and the doctors affiliated with it.

Physician's assistant: A medical practitioner (P.A.) who is specially trained to provide a basic level of diagnostic medical care, usually under the supervision of a physician.

Physician's Desk Reference (PDR): A comprehensive reference book primarily listing prescription drugs and indications for use, contraindications and dosages.

Podiatrist: A medical practitioner (D.P.M.; non-M.D., non-D.O.) who specializes in caring for feet.

Point-of-service (POS) plan: A managed-care plan in which members pay monthly premiums for which they receive all the care they need from within the network of doctors and hospitals. If the member goes outside the network for care, the insurer still pays a significant portion of the bill. Out-of-pocket costs are capped.

Preferred-provider organization (PPO): A form of managed care, similar to an HMO, usually owned by the physicians. Costs outside the network are usually not covered.

Repackaging: The purchasing of products from a pharmaceutical distributor and then repacking of them into smaller units for sale under a different label.

Residency: A post-medical school training program, usually lasting from three to five years, in which a physician completes training in a speciality area, such as anesthesiology, emergency medicine or surgery. Completion of an approved residency program is a requirement for board certification.

Second opinion: An objective evaluation, diagnosis and treatment recommendation from a medical practitioner concerning a health problem that has previously been evaluated by another medical practitioner.

Side effect: An effect of a drug or treatment that is not directly a part of the healing process.

Skilled nursing facility: An institution that offers nursing services similar to those given in a hospital, to aid recuperation of those who are seriously ill.

Specialist: A doctor who concentrates on a specific body system, age group or disorder.

Staff model: A type of HMO in which the HMO actually employs its own physicians, paying each an annual salary and possibly a bonus.

Subspecialty: A specific area of medicine within a specialty. Usually, a specialist takes one or two more years of training to develop a subspecialty.

GLOSSARY 2
Medical Abbreviations

Ah, medical abbreviations—those shorthand codes shared by doctors, pharmacists and nurses as part of a long tradition of cryptic communication that excludes consumers. Medical abbreviations are rampant in medical records and hospital charts, and they are particularly prominent when scrawled across prescription forms. Fortunately for consumers, translating those compacted terms into everyday language is not difficult. All you need is the key. To that end, we give you this table of common medical abbreviations. Note that abbreviations most likely to show up on prescription forms have been highlighted in bold.

a = before

A2 = both ears

aa. = of each

ac = before meals

Ad. = to, up to

AD = right ear

ADL = activities of daily living

ad lib = as needed, as desired

AF = auricular fibrillation

agit = shake, stir

AL = left ear

AM = morning

AMA = against medical advice

Ap. = appendicitis

Aq. = water
ASHD = arteriosclerotic heart disease
BE = barium enema
bid = twice a day
Bl. time = bleeding time
BM = bowel movement
BMR = basal metabolic rate
BP = blood pressure
BRP = bathroom privileges
Bx = biopsy
C = centigrade
c̄ = with
CA = cancer
CAD = coronary artery disease
cap(s) = capsule(s)
CBC = complete blood count
CBD = common bile duct
CC = chief complaint
cc = cubic centimeter
CCU = coronary care unit
CHD = coronary heart disease; congenital heart disease
CHF = congestive heart failure
Chol = cholesterol
Cl. time = clotting time
CNS = central nervous system
comp = compound
cont rem = continue the medicine
COPD = chronic obstructive pulmonary disease
CSF = cerebrospinal fluid
CV = cardiovascular
CVA = cerebrovascular accident
CVP = central venous pressure
CXR = chest X ray

d = give
D&C = dilation and curettage
dd in d = from day to day
dec = pour off
dexter = the right
dil = dilute
Disp. = dispense
div = divide
DM = diabetes mellitus
dos = dose
dur dolor = while pain lasts
D/W = dextrose in water
Dx = diagnosis
ECG or EKG = electrocardiogram
EEG = electroencephalogram
emp = as directed
ER = emergency room
ext = for external use
F = Fahrenheit
FBS = fasting blood sugar
febris = fever
FH = family history
Fx = fracture
GA = general anesthesia
garg = gargle
GB = gallbladder
GC = gonorrhea
GI = gastrointestinal
GL = glaucoma
gm = grams
gr = grain(s)
grad = by degrees
gravida = pregnancies

gtt = drops
GTT = glucose tolerance test
GU = genitourinary
GYN = gynecology
h = hour, hourly
HASHD = hypertensive arteriosclerotic heart disease
Hb or Hgb = hemoglobin
HCT = hematocrit
HHD = hypertensive heart disease
HOB = head of bed
HPI = history of present illness
h.s. = at bedtime
Hx = history
i = one
ii = two
iii = three
ICU = intensive care unit
I&D = incision and drainage
IM = intramuscular
I.M. = infectious mononucleosis
ind = daily
I&O = intake and output (measure fluids going into and out of body)
IPPB = intermittent positive pressure breathing
IV = intravenous
IVP = intravenous pyelogram
L = left
liq = liquid
LLE = left lower extremity
LLQ = left lower quadrant
LMP = last menstrual period
LP = lumbar puncture
LUE = left upper extremity

LUQ = left upper quadrant
Ⓜ = murmur
M = mix
m et n = morning and night
mg = milligram
MI = myocardial infarction (heart attack)
ml = milliliter
mor dict = in the manner directed
MS = mitral stenosis; morphine sulfate; multiple sclerosis
neg. = negative
N-G = nasogastric
no. = number
non rep; nr = do not repeat
NPO = non per os (nothing by mouth)
NS = normal saline
N&V = nausea and vomiting
O_2 = oxygen
o = none
$\overline{o}$ = with
ø = without
OD = right eye
O.D. = once a day
OL = left eye
OOB = out of bed
OPD = outpatient department
OR = operating room
OS = left eye
OT = occupational therapy
OU = both eyes
P; $\overline{p}$ = after
Para = number of births
Path. = pathology
pc = after meals

PE = physical examination; pulmonary embolus
PI = present illness
pil = pill
po = orally (by mouth)
Post. = posterior
post-op = postoperative, after the operation
PM = evening
PR = pulse rate
pr = by rectum
prn = as needed, as often as necessary
Prog. = prognosis
pt = patient
PT = physical therapy
PTA = prior to admission
Px = prognosis
q = every
qam = every morning
qd = daily
qh = every hour
q2h = every two hours
q3h = every three hours
q4h = every four hours
q8h = every eight hours
qhs = at hour of sleep
qid = four times a day
qn = every night
qod = every other day
qs = proper amount, quantity sufficient
qv = as much as desired
R = right
rbc = red blood cell
RBC = red blood cell count
rep = repeat

RHD = rheumatic heart disease
RLQ = right lower quadrant
RN = registered nurse
ROM = range of motion
RR = respiratory rate; recovery room
RT = radiation therapy
rub = red
RUQ = right upper quadrant
Rx = prescription; therapy
$\bar{s}$ = without
S&A = sugar and acetone (a urine test for diabetics)
sc = subcutaneous
Scop. = scopolamine
SH = social history
SICU = surgical intensive care unit
sig = write, let it be imprinted
sing = of each
sl = under the tongue
SOB = shortness of breath
sol = solution
solv = dissolve
SOP = standard operating procedure
SOS = can repeat in emergency
ss = half
SSE = soapsuds enema
stat = right away, immediately
sub Q = subcutaneous
suppos = suppository
susp = suspension
Sx = symptoms
T&A = tonsillectomy and adenoidectomy
tab(s) = tablet(s)
TAT = tetanus antitoxin

tere = rub

TIA = transient ischemic attack

tid = three times a day

tinc. or tinct. = tincture

TPR = temperature, pulse and respiration

top = apply topically

Tx = treatment

ung = ointment

ungt = ointment

URI = upper respiratory infection

ut dict = as directed

UTI = urinary tract infection

VD = venereal disease

VS = vital signs

WBC = white blood cell count

WC = wheelchair

YO = year old

x = times

↑ = increase

↗ = increasing

↓ = decrease

↙ = decreasing

→ = leads to

← = resulting from

♂ = male

♀ = female

PART II

DIAL 800 FOR HEALTH

HOW TO USE THIS DIRECTORY

Dial 800 for Health is like having your own personal health-care researcher to provide you with the answers and information you need to make important health-care decisions. On the following pages, specific conditions and services are listed alphabetically in major headings. By turning to a particular condition or service, you will find the organizations and agencies that can help you. Included for each organization are the name, address, toll-free telephone number, hours of operation and type of information or service provided.

The index and subject cross-reference found in the back of the book can also help you to locate an agency or organization. For example, if you want information on Crohn's disease and you didn't find it listed among the major headings, turn to the index and subject cross-reference and locate Crohn's disease, which then directs you to the section on digestive diseases.

Types of Toll-Free Numbers

This edition of *Dial 800 for Health* includes listings within the new *888* toll-free telephone exchange, which was added when the supply of toll-free *800* numbers was exhausted. Most of the toll-free telephone numbers listed in this directory are accessible from every state. Just dial *1 + 800* (or *888) + the number.* However, the telephone numbers of some organizations such as poison control centers are accessible only from a single state, portions of a state or a city. For example, the listing for the Poison Center in Omaha, Nebraska, which can be accessed only from Nebraska and Wyoming, is listed:

The Poison Center
Omaha, NE
800-955-9119 Nebraska and Wyoming

You will also find organizations that have two separate toll-free numbers—one for national use and the other for use in a specific state—as in the following example:

Shriners Hospital Referral Line
Tampa, FL
800-237-5055
800-282-9161 Florida

Some organizations have both a toll-free number and a long-distance (unless, of course, you are calling from within the local area of the number) number listed. This is done in the event that the toll-free number is busy or out of service. These listings appear as follows:

Neurofibromatosis
Lanham, MD
800-942-6825
301-577-8984

Several organizations use their names, initials or another mnemonic device as part of their telephone numbers. In these cases, we have listed both the mnemonic device and the numeric translation to make it easier to dial, as in the following example:

American International Hospital Cancer Program
Zion, IL
800-FOR-HELP (800-367-4357)

Callers who require services for the hearing- or speech-impaired will find numbers identified by TDD (for use with telecommunications devices) and TTY (for use with teletype devices), as in the following example:

AIDS Hotline
Research Triangle Park, NC
800-243-7889 TDD

The final type of toll-free number found in this directory is the Spanish language line. Some organizations have a dedicated Spanish line, while others offer Spanish on a separate extension, as in the following example:

AIDS Hotline
Research Triangle Park, NC
800-344-7432 Spanish

Hours of operation are listed in local time zones, either eastern, central, mountain or Pacific. There are no references to daylight savings time. Also, many of these organizations are staffed by volunteers who answer the telephone from their homes. Therefore, unless otherwise specified, please be considerate by calling during regular business hours, generally 9:00 A.M. to 5:00 P.M. If you're unsure of the time zone, check the state location on a time zone map, which may be found in your local telephone directory.

With the tremendous growth of on-line services and in-home computers, we've added the e-mail addresses of many organizations. However, be aware that in some cases you may be charged for access to these on-line services, thereby defeating the purpose of toll-free dialing.

Every toll-free number listed in this directory was verified just prior to publication and found to be in operation. However, should you encounter a problem dialing any of the *800* or *888* numbers, we suggest that you call the toll-free directory assistance operator at 800-555-1212.

A brief explanation that describes the type of service or information provided by the organization follows each listing. This will help you to determine whether the organization does indeed provide the kind of information you desire.

The People's Medical Society makes no claims or

guarantees for the organizations listed in this directory. *Dial 800 for Health* is not an endorsement or recommendation of these organizations by the People's Medical Society. We cannot be responsible for the services offered or the content of the information provided. As always, we encourage you to exercise your own good judgment when contacting any of these groups.

ADOPTION

AASK America
657 Mission St., Suite 601
San Francisco, CA 94105
800-232-2751

Provides information on how to adopt children with special needs such as those with mental and physical disabilities.

Child Reach
155 Plan Way
Warwick, RI 02886
800-556-7918
8:45 A.M. to 8:45 P.M. (eastern time), Monday to Friday

Provides information on how to become a sponsor to a child living in the Third World.

Concerned United Birthparents
2000 Walker St.
Des Moines, IA 50317
800-822-2777
515-263-9558 Iowa
24 hours a day, seven days a week

Provides information on support groups designed for birth parents who gave up their children for adoption and are now seeking to come to terms with their decision. Also makes referrals to support groups in the caller's area.

Edna Gladney Center
2300 Hemphill St.
Ft. Worth, TX 76110
800-433-2922
800-772-2740 Texas
8:30 A.M. to 5:00 P.M. (central time), Monday to Saturday

Provides counseling and shelter to single pregnant women who want to place their children for adoption. Information packet available upon request.

International Children's Care
2711 N.E. 134th St.
Vancouver, WA 98686
800-422-7729

Provides information to couples or individuals who are interested in international adoptions. Counsels prospective parents on the adoption and immigration laws of the foreign country.

National Adoption Center
1500 Walnut St.
Philadelphia, PA 19102
800-862-3678
215-925-0200 Philadelphia
9:00 A.M. to 5:00 P.M. (eastern time), Monday to Friday
Provides adoption information concerning hard-to-place children and children with special needs.

Pregnancy Counseling Services
Liberty Godparent Home
Fort Early Building
11 Oakridge Blvd., Suite 201
Lynchburg, VA 24501
800-542-4453
804-384-3043 Virginia
24 hours a day, seven days a week
Provides information on residential programs for unwed mothers. Offers counseling and adoption services. Also makes referrals to support groups in the caller's area.

AEROBIC EXERCISE

Aerobic and Fitness Association of America
15250 Ventura Blvd., Suite 310
Sherman Oaks, CA 91403
800-446-2322
800-445-5950
800-343-2584 California
800-225-2322 Canada and Mexico
8:30 A.M. to 5:00 P.M. (Pacific time), Monday to Friday
Provides basic information on aerobic exercise, certified instructors and prevention and treatment of aerobics-related injuries.

National Dance-Exercise Instructors Training Association
1503 S. Washington Ave., Suite 208
Minneapolis, MN 55454
800-237-6242
612-340-1306 Minnesota
Provides information on aerobics instructors and seminars nationwide.

AIDS
(Acquired Immune Deficiency Syndrome)

AIDS Clinical Trials Information Service
P.O. Box 6421
Rockville, MD 20849–6421
800-874-2572
800-243-7012 TTY
9:00 A.M. to 7:00 P.M. (eastern time), Monday to Friday
e-mail: Actis@cdcnac.aspensys.com

Provides information on the status of federally and privately sponsored experimental drug trials for human immunodeficiency virus (HIV) and AIDS. Information packet available upon request.

AIDS Hotline
c/o American Social Health Association
P.O. Box 13827
Research Triangle Park, NC 27709
800-342-2437
800-243-7889 TDD
24 hours a day, seven days a week
800-344-7432 Spanish
8:00 A.M. to 2:00 A.M. (eastern time), seven days a week

Provides information on human immunodeficiency virus (HIV) and AIDS transmission and prevention. Answers specific questions concerning HIV and AIDS. Also makes referrals for testing and counseling. Information packet available upon request.

American Academy of Pediatrics
Pediatric AIDS Coalition
601 13th St., NW, Suite 400N
Washington, DC 20005
800-336-5475
202-662-7460 District of Columbia
9:00 A.M. to 5:00 P.M. (eastern time), Monday to Friday

Provides information on AIDS education programs for adults and children in churches, schools and other community organizations.

Haitian AIDS Hotline
8037 N.E. Second Ave.
Miami, FL 33138
800-722-7432
8:30 A.M. to 5:00 P.M. (eastern time), Monday to Friday

Provides human immunodeficiency virus (HIV) and AIDS information specifically tailored to the Haitian population.

Multicultural Training Resource Center
1540 Market St., Suite 320
San Francisco, CA 94102
800-545-6642 California

Provides human immunodeficiency virus (HIV) and AIDS information specifically targeted to diverse cultural groups.

Names Project
2362 Market St.
P.O. Box 14573
San Francisco, CA 94114
800-872-6263 California
415-863-5511
9:00 A.M. to 6:00 P.M. (Pacific time), Monday to Friday

Provides information on how to add names to the AIDS Memorial Quilt, which commemorates those men, women and children who have lost their lives to AIDS.

National AIDS Information Clearinghouse
P.O. Box 6003
Rockville, MD 20849–6003
800-458-5231
9:00 A.M. to 7:00 P.M. (eastern time), Monday to Friday

Provides recorded messages in English and Spanish with information on organizational and educational materials, clinical drug trials and how to order publications.

National Native American AIDS Prevention Center
3515 Grand Ave., Suite 100
Oakland, CA 94610
800-283-2437
8:30 A.M. to 5:00 P.M. (Pacific time), Monday to Friday
510-444-2051 Oakland

Provides referrals to Native Americans regarding counseling and testing centers. Information packet available upon request.

People With AIDS Coalition
31 W. 26th St.
New York, NY 10010
800-828-3280
212-532-0290
10:00 A.M. to 6:00 P.M. (eastern time), Monday to Friday
1:00 P.M. to 5:00 P.M. (eastern time), Saturday and Sunday

Provides information and referral services to callers. Also provides publications in both English and Spanish.

Project Inform
220 Market St.
San Francisco, CA 94103
800-822-7422
800-334-7422 California
10:00 A.M. to 4:00 P.M. (Pacific time), Monday to Friday
10:00 A.M. to 1:00 P.M. (Pacific time), Saturday
Answering machine at all other times

Provides current information on treatment options for persons with human immunodefiency virus (HIV) and AIDS, as well as information on organizations that provide the treatments. Also operates an outreach and advocacy program.

Teens Teaching AIDS Prevention
3030 Walnut St.
Kansas City, MO 64108
800-234-8336
816-561-8784 Kansas City
4:00 P.M. to 8:00 P.M. (central time), Monday to Friday
Answering machine at all other times

Provides information and counseling on human immunodeficiency virus (HIV) and AIDS from a teen's perspective. Makes referrals to AIDS organizations and other resources. Some literature available at a nominal charge.

ALLERGIES AND ASTHMA

Allergy and Asthma Network/Mothers of Asthmatics
3554 Chain Bridge Rd., Suite 200
Fairfax, VA 22030
800-878-4403
9:00 A.M. to 5:00 P.M. (eastern time), Monday to Friday

Provides patient education and information on asthma and allergy. Sells publications and videos. Individual membership ($25) includes subscription to the MA Report, *a monthly newsletter.*

Allergy Information Referral Line
American Academy of Allergy and Immunology
611 E. Wells St.
Milwaukee, WI 53202
800-822-2762
414-272-6071 Wisconsin
8:00 A.M. to 5:00 P.M. (central time), Monday to Friday

Provides information on the diagnosis and treatment of allergies and asthma. Also makes referrals to allergy specialists.

American College of Allergy and Immunology
800 W. Northwest Hwy., Suite 1080
Palatine, IL 60067
800-842-7777
24 hours a day, Monday to Friday

Provides information on various allergies and the treatment options available.

Asthma and Allergy Foundation of America
1125 15th St., NW, Suite 502
Washington, DC 20005
800-727-8462
202-466-7643 District of Columbia

Provides U.S. maps showing zones where plants are likely to cause allergy problems. Also provides educational materials on asthma and allergies.

The Food Allergy Network
10400 Eaton Pl., Suite 107
Fairfax, VA 22030–2208
800-929-4040
9:00 A.M. to 5:00 P.M. (eastern time), Monday to Friday

Provides information on, and works to increase public awareness of, food allergies. Individual membership ($24) includes a subscription to the bimonthly newsletter Food Allergy News *and consumer alerts.*

National Jewish Asthma Center
1400 Jackson St.
Denver, CO 80206
800-222-5864
303-398-1477 Denver
8:00 A.M. to 5:00 P.M. (mountain time), Monday to Friday

Answers questions about asthma, emphysema, chronic bronchitis and other respiratory diseases. Also makes referrals to doctors in the caller's area. Information packet available upon request.

ALZHEIMER'S DISEASE

Alzheimer's Association
919 N. Michigan Ave., Suite 1000
Chicago, IL 60611
800-272-3900
8:30 A.M. to 5:00 P.M. (central time), Monday to Friday
Answering machine at all other times
e-mail: Info@alz.org

Provides information on Alzheimer's disease and related disorders. Also makes referrals to chapters in the caller's area.

Alzheimer's Disease Education and Referral Center
National Institute on Aging
Public Information Office
Building 31, Room 5C27
Bethesda, MD 20892
800-438-4380
8:30 A.M. to 5:00 P.M. (eastern time), Monday to Friday
Answering machine at all other times

Provides information on Alzheimer's disease to the public. Also provides information for health professionals. Information packet available upon request.

American Health Assistance Foundation
15825 Shady Grove Rd., Suite 140
Rockville, MD 20850
800-437-2423
301-948-3244 Maryland
9:00 A.M. to 5:00 P.M. (eastern time), Monday to Friday

Provides public education materials on Alzheimer's relief programs and provides funding for such programs. Also provides financial assistance to families in need of relief services.

National Family Caregivers Association
9621 Bexhill Dr.
Kensington, MD 20895–3104
800-896-3650
301-942-6430
9:00 A.M. to 5:00 P.M. (eastern time), Monday to Friday

Provides information and offers support and counseling to individuals who find themselves faced with the responsibility of providing care to a family member.

AMYOTROPHIC LATERAL SCLEROSIS (ALS; "Lou Gehrig's Disease")

ALS Association
21021 Ventura Blvd., Suite 321
Woodland Hills, CA 91364
800-782-4747
818-340-7500 San Fernando Valley
8:00 A.M. to 5:00 P.M. (Pacific time), Monday to Friday

Provides education, information and referral services to ALS patients and their families. Also makes referrals to chapters in the caller's area.

ANEMIA

Aplastic Anemia Foundation of America
P.O. Box 22689
Baltimore, MD 21203
800-747-2820
410-955-2803 Maryland
9:00 A.M. to 5:00 P.M. (eastern time), Monday to Friday

Provides information and counseling to people with aplastic anemia.

National Association for Sickle Cell Disease
3345 Wilshire Blvd., Suite 1106
Los Angeles, CA 90010–1880
800-421-8453
213-736-5455 Los Angeles
8:30 A.M. to 5:00 P.M. (Pacific time), Monday to Friday

Provides materials, trains counselors and offers programs to medical professionals and the public. Also supports research, conducts public education campaigns and provides diagnostic screening.

ARTHRITIS

Arthritis Consulting Services
4620 N. State Road 7, Suite 206
Ft. Lauderdale, FL 33319
800-327-3027
8:30 A.M. to 4:00 P.M. (eastern time), Monday to Friday

Provides information on holistic approaches to treating arthritis.

Arthritis Foundation Information Line
P.O. Box 19000
Atlanta, GA 30326
800-283-7800
404-872-7100 Georgia
9:00 A.M. to 7:00 P.M. (eastern time), Monday to Friday

Provides physician referrals and information concerning chapters in the caller's area. Information packet available upon request.

Spondylitis Association of America
P.O. Box 5872
Sherman Oaks, CA 92413
800-777-8189
818-981-1616
8:00 A.M. to 5:00 P.M. (Pacific time), Monday to Friday
Answering machine at all other times
e-mail: info@spondylitis.org

Provides information on the diagnosis and treatment of the condition. Also makes referrals to support groups in the caller's area. Information packet available upon request.

BEHÇET'S SYNDROME

American Behçet's Association
P.O. Box 27494
Tempe, AZ 85285–7494
800-723-4238
10:00 A.M. to 8:00 P.M. (eastern time), Monday to Friday
e-mail: NYYY49C@Prodigy.com

Provides information on this condition to patients and their families. Also provides mutual support and meets on Prodigy (an on-line computer service).

BIRTH-RELATED DISORDERS

American Cleft Palate Educational Foundation
1218 Grandview Ave.
Pittsburgh, PA 15211
800-24-CLEFT (800-242-5338)
800-232-5338 Pennsylvania
7:30 A.M. to 4:30 P.M. (eastern time), Monday to Friday
Answering machine at all other times

Provides parents with information on feeding techniques and proper dental care for children with cleft palates. Also makes referrals to support groups in the caller's area. Information packet available upon request.

Anencephaly Research and Help Line
128 W. Woodstock Circle
Spring, TX 77381
888-206-7526
24 hours a day, seven days a week

Provides information and support services to parents with children who were born anencephalic.

Association of Birth Defect Children
827 Irma St.
Orlando, FL 32803
800-313-2232
407-245-7035
24 hours a day, seven days a week

Provides support services to parents of children with birth defects or developmental disabilities. Maintains birth defects registry that tracks birth defects that may be related to chemical, radiation or other environmental factors. Also operates a referral service that links parents in a support network.

Autism Society of America
7910 Woodmont Ave., Suite 650
Bethesda, MD 20814
800-328-8476
301-657-0881
9:00 A.M. to 5:00 P.M. (eastern time), Monday to Friday

Provides information on the diagnosis and treatment of autism. Promotes public awareness and understanding of adults and children with autism.

Batten's Disease Support and Research Association
2600 Parsons Ave.
Columbus, OH 43207
800-448-4570
614-445-4161
24 hours a day, seven days a week

Provides information and support to families of children afflicted with Batten's disease. Also makes referrals to support groups in the caller's area.

Beckwith-Wiedemann Syndrome Support Network
3206 Braeburn Circle
Ann Arbor, MI 48108
800-837-2976
313-973-0263
9:00 A.M. to 5:00 P.M. (eastern time), Monday to Friday
Answering machine at all other times

Provides information and assistance to families of children with Beckwith-Wiedemann syndrome. Also promotes research into the causes, early diagnosis and treatment of the condition.

Cornelia de Lange Syndrome (CdLS) Foundation
60 Dyer Ave.
Collinsville, CT 06022
800-223-8355
800-753-2357 Canada
9:00 A.M. to 4:30 P.M. (eastern time), Monday to Friday
Answering machine at all other times

Provides general information on the birth defects caused by CdLS. Also operates a support system for parents and makes referrals to chapters in the caller's area. Information packet available upon request.

Cystic Fibrosis Foundation
6931 Arlington Rd.
Bethesda, MD 20814
800-344-4823
301-951-4422
8:30 A.M. to 5:30 P.M. (eastern time), Monday to Friday

Provides information on cystic fibrosis. Also makes referrals to hospital treatment centers and support groups in the caller's area. Information packet available upon request.

Cystinosis Foundation
1212 Broadway
Oakland, CA 94612
800-392-8458
510-235-1052

Provides information on the genetic disorder cystinosis and helps to raise funds for research. Also provides support to parents of children with this condition.

Fragile X Syndrome
1441 York St., #215
Denver, CO 80206
800-688-8765
303-333-6155
9:00 A.M. to 5:00 P.M. (mountain time), Monday to Friday
Answering machine at all other times

Provides information on the detection and treatment of the hereditary condition fragile X syndrome. Also provides information on support networks and makes referrals in the caller's area.

International Rett Syndrome Association
9121 Piscataway Rd., #2B
Clinton, MD 20735–2561
800-818-7388
301-856-3334
9:00 A.M. to 5:00 P.M. (eastern time), Monday to Friday
e-mail: irsa@paltech.com

Provides information and counseling to parents with children afflicted with Rett syndrome. Also promotes and supports research efforts.

National Down Syndrome Congress
1800 Dempster St.
Park Ridge, IL 60068
800-232-6372
9:00 A.M. to 5:00 P.M. (central time), Monday to Friday

Provides information and referrals on Down syndrome. Publishes a newsletter and sponsors an annual convention.

National Down Syndrome Society
666 Broadway
New York, NY 10012
800-221-4602
9:00 A.M. to 5:00 P.M. (eastern time), Monday to Friday
Answering machine at all other times

Makes referrals to support groups in the caller's area. Publications available for a small fee. Information packet available upon request.

National Gaucher Disease Foundation
11140 Rockville Pike, #350
Rockville, MD 20852–3106
800-925-8885
9:00 A.M. to 5:00 P.M. (eastern time), Monday to Friday
Answering machine at all other times

Provides information and assistance to families with children suffering from Gaucher disease. Also makes referrals to treatment centers and support groups in the caller's area.

Prader-Willi Syndrome Association
2510 S. Brentwood Blvd., #220
St. Louis, MO 63144
800-926-4797
314-962-7644
8:00 A.M. to 4:00 P.M. (central time), Monday to Friday
Answering machine at all other times
e-mail: pwsausa@aol.com

Provides information and support service to parents of children with Prader-Willi syndrome. Information packet available upon request.

Spina Bifida Association of America
4590 MacArthur Blvd., NW, Suite 250
Washington, DC 20007
800-621-3141
301-770-7222 Maryland
9:00 A.M. to 5:00 P.M. (eastern time), Monday to Friday
Answering machine at all other times

Provides information on the birth defect spina bifida. Also makes referrals to chapters in the caller's area.

Sturge-Weber Foundation
P.O. Box 418
Mt. Freedom, NJ 07970
800-627-5482
8:30 A.M. to 2:30 P.M. (eastern time), Monday to Thursday
Answering machine at all other times

Provides information on Sturge-Weber syndrome. Operates a mutual support network for families affected by this condition. Also makes referrals in the caller's area. Information packet available upon request.

Tay-Sachs Foundation
1303 Paper Mill Rd.
Erdenheim, PA 19038
800-672-2022
9:00 A.M. to 5:00 P.M. (eastern time), Monday to Friday
e-mail: 72624.3502E@Compuserve.com

Provides information on Tay-Sachs disease as well as advocacy and support for families with children affected by this genetic condition. Also makes referrals to support groups in the caller's area.

Turner's Syndrome Society
814 Glencarin Ave.
Toronto, Ontario
Canada M6B 2A3
800-465-6744
416-781-2086
24 hours a day, seven days a week

Provides information and support to families affected by Turner's syndrome. Also makes referrals to Canadian and U.S. support groups in the caller's area.

Turner's Syndrome Society of the United States
1313 S.E. Fifth St., Suite 327
Minneapolis, MN 55414
800-365-9944
612-379-3607
8:30 A.M. to 5:00 P.M. (central time), Monday to Friday
e-mail: Tesch005@tc.umn.edu

Provides information on Turner's syndrome. Also works to increase public awareness and support for research into the causes and prevention of this genetic disorder affecting females. Information packet available upon request.

United Cerebral Palsy Association
1522 K St., NW, Suite 1112
Washington, DC 20005
800-872-5827
202-842-1266
9:00 A.M. to 5:00 P.M. (eastern time), Monday to Friday

Provides information on the diagnosis and treatment of cerebral palsy. Works to establish local programs that help people with the disease move into mainstream society.

BLOOD DISORDERS

National Hemophilia Foundation
110 Greene St., Suite 303
New York, NY 10012
800-424-2634
212-431-8541
9:00 A.M. to 5:00 P.M. (eastern time), Monday to Friday
Answering machine at all other times

Provides information and referrals to families affected by hemophilia. Also supports research and disseminates information to raise the public awareness about hemophilia.

National Marrow Donor Program
3433 Broadway St., NE, Suite 400
Minneapolis, MN 55413–1762
800-654-1247 Extension 149 for Spanish
8:00 A.M. to 6:00 P.M. (central time), Monday to Friday
Answering machine at all other times

Maintains a registry of bone marrow donors. Also provides information on how interested individuals can become active in the registry program.

BURN CARE

Phoenix Society
National Organization for Burn Survivors
11 Rust Hill Rd.
Levittown, PA 19056
800-888-2876
215-946-4788

Provides information on the self-help services available to burn victims and their families. Helps burn victims deal with their trauma and provides the psychological support they need to return to normal lives and interests. Information packet available upon request.

Shriners Hospital Referral Line
2900 Rocky Point Dr.
Tampa, FL 33607–1435
800-237-5055
800-282-9161 Florida
8:00 A.M. to 5:00 P.M. (eastern time), Monday to Friday
Provides information on burn treatment programs available at Shriners hospitals.

CANCER

AMC Cancer Information and Counseling Line
American Medical Center
1600 Pierce St.
Denver, CO 80214
800-525-3777
303-233-6501 Denver
8:30 A.M. to 4:45 P.M. (mountain time), Monday to Friday
Provides the latest information on cancer prevention, detection and treatment methods. Offers counseling. Also makes referrals to support groups in the caller's area.

American Association of Oral and Maxillofacial Surgeons
9700 Bryn Mawr Ave.
Rosemont, IL 60018
800-467-5268
8:30 A.M. to 5:00 P.M. (central time), Monday to Friday
Answering machine at all other times
Provides information on oral cancer. Also makes referrals to oral surgeons in the caller's area.

American Brain Tumor Association
2720 River Rd., Suite 146
Des Plaines, IL 60018
800-886-2282
847-827-9910
e-mail: ABTA@aol.com
Provides information on brain tumors and support groups in the caller's area. Encourages and supports research efforts aimed at treating brain tumors.

American Cancer Society
1599 Clifton Rd., NE
Atlanta, GA 30329
800-227-2345
8:30 A.M. to 4:30 P.M. (eastern time), Monday to Friday

Provides general information on the society's programs and services. Makes referrals to chapters in the caller's area. Also answers questions about cancer, including those regarding prevention, diagnosis, treatment and rehabilitation.

American International Hospital Cancer Program
2501 Emmaus Ave.
Zion, IL 60099
800-FOR-HELP (800-367-4357)
708-872-4561

Provides information on cancer treatment programs available at hospitals.

Cancer Care
1180 Avenue of the Americas
New York, NY 10036
800-813-4673 Extension 2 for Spanish
e-mail: info@cancercareinc.org

Provides information and counseling to cancer patients and their families. Also makes referrals to support groups in the caller's area.

Cancer Research Institute
681 Fifth Ave.
New York, NY 10022
800-992-2623
9:00 A.M. to 5:00 P.M. (eastern time), Monday to Friday
Answering machine at all other times
e-mail: info@cancerresearch.org

Provides information on recent developments in the diagnosis, treatment and prevention of cancer.

Candlelighters Childhood Cancer Foundation
7910 Woodmont Ave., Suite 460
Bethesda, MD 20814
800-366-2223
24 hours a day, seven days a week

Provides information and services such as a 24-hour crisis line and transportation to families of childhood cancer patients. Serves as a clearinghouse and liaison between parents and medical professionals. Establishes Ronald McDonald houses, where family members of patients may stay while the patient undergoes treatment.

CHEMOcare
231 North Ave., W
Westfield, NJ 07090
800-55-CHEMO (800-552-4366)
908-233-1103 New Jersey
9:00 A.M. to 5:30 P.M. (eastern time), Monday to Friday
Answering machine at all other times
e-mail: chemocare@aol.com

Provides information and support to cancer patients who are currently undergoing chemotherapy or radiation therapy. Operates a one-on-one emotional support network for these patients.

Comprehensive Cancer Center
University of Alabama at Birmingham
University Station
Birmingham, AL 35294
800-UAB-0933 (800-822-0933)
205-934-5077

Provides information on cancer treatment programs available at the university center.

International Cancer Alliance
4853 Cordell Ave., Suite 11
Bethesda, MD 20814
800-422-7361
9:00 A.M. to 5:00 P.M. (eastern time), Monday to Friday
Answering machine at all other times

Provides free information on various types of cancers, including diagnostic tests, staging and treatments. Also publishes quarterly reports on progress against cancer.

International Myeloma Foundation
2120 Stanley Hills Dr.
Los Angeles, CA 90046
800-452-2873
213-654-3023
8:00 A.M. to 5:00 P.M. (Pacific time), Monday to Friday
Answering machine at all other times
e-mail: TheIMF@aol.com

Provides information to patients and professionals on the diagnosis and treatment of myeloma. Supports research and sponsors conferences. Also publishes a quarterly newsletter.

Leukemia Society of America
600 Third Ave.
New York, NY 10016
800-955-4572
212-573-8484
24 hours a day, seven days a week

Provides information on the latest research into the causes and treatment of leukemia and related cancers. Also sponsors national programs on patient and professional education.

Make Today Count
Mid-American Cancer Center
1235 E. Cherokee St.
Springfield, MO 65804–2263
800-432-2273
417-885-2000
9:00 A.M. to 4:30 P.M. (central time), Monday to Friday
Answering machine at all other times

Provides information on this mutual support organization, that helps people affected by life-threatening illnesses to lead full and complete lives. Encourages mutual support and self-help.

Mathews Foundation for Prostate Cancer Research
817 Commons Dr.
Sacramento, CA 95825
800-234-6284
916-567-1400
e-mail: mathews@sna.com

Provides information on the symptoms, diagnosis and treatment of prostate cancer. Also responds to individual questions concerning the effects of the disease.

National Alliance of Breast Cancer Organizations
9 E. 37th St., 10th Floor
New York, NY 10016
800-719-9154
24 hours a day, seven days a week
e-mail: NABCOinfo@aol.com

Provides information on breast cancer. Also serves as an advocate for legislation and regulatory concerns of breast cancer patients and their families.

National Brain Tumor Foundation
785 Market St., Suite 1600
San Francisco, CA 94103
800-934-2873
415-284-0208
9:00 A.M. to 5:00 P.M. (Pacific time), Monday to Friday
Answering machine at all other times

Provides information on the latest research into discovering an effective treatment for brain tumors. Also makes referrals to support groups in the caller's area.

National Cancer Institute
Cancer Information Service
9000 Rockville Pike, Suite 414
Bethesda, MD 20892
800-422-6237
800-638-6070 Alaska
800-524-1234 Hawaii
9:00 A.M. to 10:00 P.M. (eastern time), Monday to Friday

Provides information on various types of cancers and the latest treatments available for those cancers. Information packets in both English and Spanish available upon request.

Nutrition Hotline
American Institute for Cancer Research
1759 R St., NW
Washington, DC 20009
800-843-8114
202-328-7744 District of Columbia
9:00 A.M. to 9:00 P.M. (eastern time), Monday to Thursday
9:00 A.M. to 5:00 P.M. (eastern time), Friday
Answering machine at all other times

Provides information on the role of diet and nutrition in cancer prevention and how nutrition may be used to assist a cancer treatment program. Also responds to specific requests for information.

The Skin Cancer Foundation
P.O. Box 561
New York, NY 10156
800-754-6490
212-725-5176
24 hours a day, seven days a week

Provides educational materials on skin cancer. Also conducts seminars to help reduce the incidence of skin cancer.

Susan G. Komen Breast Cancer Foundation
5005 LBJ Freeway, Suite 370
Dallas, TX 75244
800-462-9273
24 hours a day, seven days a week

Provides information on general breast health, including information on breast cancer. Supports events that raise money to research the causes of breast cancer. Also makes referrals to chapters in the caller's area.

Y-ME
National Breast Cancer Organization
212 W. Van Buren, 5th Floor
Chicago, IL 60607
800-221-2141
24 hours a day, seven days a week
800-986-9505 Spanish
9:00 A.M. to 5:00 P.M. (central time), Monday to Friday

Provides information and support to women undergoing treatment for breast cancer. Also provides information on prostheses after breast surgery.

CHILDREN'S SERVICES

American Academy of Pediatrics
P.O. Box 927
141 N.W. Point Blvd.
Elk Grove, IL 60007
800-433-9016
800-421-0589 Illinois

Provides information on pediatric care and the role of the pediatrician.

American Association for Protecting Children
Division of American Humane Association
63 Inverness Dr., E
Englewood, CO 80112
800-227-5242
303-792-9900 Colorado
8:30 A.M. to 5:00 P.M. (mountain time), Monday to Friday
Answering machine at all other times

Provides services to professionals who work in the child protection field. Also conducts research and program evaluations of child welfare agencies. Information packet available upon request.

Boystown Hotline
Father Flanagan's Boystown
Boystown, NE 68010
800-448-3000
24 hours a day, seven days a week

Provides assistance to runaway and homeless children regardless of race, color or creed.

Child Find Hotline
P.O. Box 277
New Paltz, NY 12561
800-426-5678
914-255-1848 New York
24 hours a day, seven days a week

Operates an international locator service for missing and abducted children. Also maintains a registry of missing children.

Children's Defense Fund
122 C St., NW, Suite 400
Washington, DC 20001
800-CDF-1200 (800-233-1200)
202-628-8787 District of Columbia
9:00 A.M. to 5:00 P.M. (eastern time), Monday to Friday

Provides information on the expanding field of children's rights as recognized by law and is involved in social and educational programs affecting children. Information packet available upon request.

Children's Wish Foundation
7840 Roswell Rd., Suite 301
Atlanta, GA 30350
800-323-9474
404-393-9474 Georgia
9:00 A.M. to 5:00 P.M. (eastern time), Monday to Friday

Provides information on programs that seek to grant a dying child his or her final wish. Works with organizations and individuals who want to become Wish Foundation supporters.

Covenant House
460 W. 41st St.
New York, NY 10036
800-999-9999
24 hours a day, seven days a week

Provides assistance to runaways and homeless youth. Also provides temporary shelter until the child's situation at home can be resolved.

Feingold Association of the United States
P.O. Box 6550
Alexandria, VA 22306
800-321-3287
24 hours a day, seven days a week

Provides information on the Feingold Program, which uses diet to treat children with learning and behavioral problems. Also makes referrals to support groups in the caller's area. Information packet available upon request.

Human Growth Foundation
7777 Leesburg Pike
Falls Church, VA 22043
800-451-6434
703-883-1773
8:30 A.M. to 5:00 P.M. (eastern time), Monday to Friday
Answering machine at all other times

Makes referrals to chapters on growth disorders in the caller's area. Information packets available upon request.

Informed Parents Against VAPP (vaccine-associated paralytic polio)
P.O. Box 53212
Washington, DC 20009
888-363-8277

Provides information to families who have been affected by vaccine-associated paralytic polio as a result of immunization. Helps parents network and exchange information.

"Just Say No" Kids Club International
2101 Webster St., Suite 1300
Oakland, CA 94612
800-258-2766
510-939-6666

Provides information on drug prevention programs for children and on how to start a "Just Say No" chapter.

Kevin Collins Foundation for Missing Children
P.O. Box 590473
San Francisco, CA 94159
800-272-0012

Provides counseling and education to the families of missing or abducted children and helps them through the ordeal.

Kidsrights
10100 Park Cedar Dr.
Charlotte, NC 28210
800-892-5437
8:30 A.M. to 5:00 P.M. (eastern time), Monday to Friday

Provides information to parents and other interested individuals on how to establish programs that work to combat teen suicide.

Little People of America
7238 Piedmont Dr.
Dallas, TX 75227–9324
800-24-DWARF (800-243-9273)
214-388-9576
9:00 A.M. to 5:00 P.M. (central time), Monday to Friday

Provides information and support to children, teens and young adults who are vertically challenged. Promotes fellowship and an exchange of ideas on how to cope with physical and emotional problems.

Missing Children Awareness Foundation
13094 95th St., N
Largo, FL 34643
800-741-7233

Provides assistance and referrals to parents of missing children.

Missing Children Help Center
410 Ware Blvd., Suite 400
Tampa, FL 33619
800-872-5437

Provides assistance to parents of missing children by publicizing the children's photographs in newspapers, brochures and flyers.

National Association for the Education of Young Children
1834 Connecticut Ave., NW
Washington, DC 20009
800-424-2460
9:00 A.M. to 5:00 P.M. (eastern time), Monday to Friday

Provides information and referrals to accredited child-care programs.

National Child Watch Campaign
P.O. Box 1368
Jackson, MI 49204
800-222-1464

Provides information on child safety and how to establish a child-watch program to protect children from being kidnapped. Also provides counseling and support services to parents whose children have been kidnapped or are missing.

National Hotline for Missing and Exploited Children
2101 Wilson Blvd., Suite 550
Arlington, VA 22201
800-843-5678
7:30 A.M. to 11:00 P.M. (eastern time), Monday to Friday
10:00 A.M. to 6:00 P.M. (eastern time), Saturday

Operates a hotline for reporting sightings of missing children and children exploited by crime, prostitution and pornography. Provides technical assistance to legal authorities in the hunt for missing or kidnapped children.

National Information Clearinghouse for Infants With Disabilities and Life-Threatening Conditions
University of South Carolina
Benson Building, 1st Floor
Columbia, SC 29208
800-922-9234 Voice and TDD
800-922-1107 Voice and TDD South Carolina
9:00 A.M. to 5:00 P.M. (eastern time), Monday to Friday
Answering machine at all other times

Provides information to families with children who have rare or life-threatening conditions. Also offers referrals to professional and community services in the caller's area. Offers special services to Vietnam veterans and their families.

National Resource Center on Child Sexual Abuse
107 Lincoln St.
Huntsville, AL 35801
800-543-7006

Provides resources to agencies dealing with children who have been sexually abused. Also provides bibliographies and articles on the sexual abuse of children.

National Runaway Hotline
Office of the Governor
P.O. Box 12428
Austin, TX 78711
800-231-6946
800-392-3352 Texas

Provides assistance to runaway children by making referrals to shelters and other agencies. Also delivers messages to the families of runaway children.

National Runaway Switchboard
3080 N. Lincoln Ave.
Chicago, IL 60657
800-621-4000
24 hours a day, seven days a week

Provides counseling and referrals to runaway youths 18 years of age and younger.

Operation Lookout
National Center for Missing Youth
P.O. Box 231
Mount Lake Terrace, WA 98043
800-782-7335

Provides assistance in locating missing children.

Parent Help Line
Nashua Brookside Hospital
11 Northwest Blvd.
Nashua, NH 03063
800-543-6381

Provides referrals to organizations that can aid parents in obtaining treatment and counseling for troubled children.

Shriners Hospital Referral Line
2900 Rocky Point Dr.
Tampa, FL 33607–1435
800-237-5055
800-282-9161 Florida
8:00 A.M. to 5:00 P.M. (eastern time), Monday to Friday

Provides information on children's services available at Shriners hospitals.

Teen Crisis Hotline
498 S. Spring St.
Crestview, FL 32536
800-262-8336 Florida

Provides information and referrals to teenagers facing crises in their lives.

Toughlove International
P.O. Box 1069
Doylestown, PA 18901
800-333-1069
215-348-7090 Pennsylvania

Serves as a support group for parents of teenage children with behavioral problems. Makes referrals in both the United States and Canada.

Vanished Children's Alliance
1407 Parkmoor Ave., Suite 200
San Jose, CA 95126
800-826-4743
408-971-4822
24 hours a day, seven days a week

Provides information on missing and recovered children.

Youth Crisis Hotline
10225 Ulmerton Rd., Suite 4-A
Largo, FL 34641
800-442-4673

Provides information on child abuse. Also serves as an advocacy group for abused children.

CHRONIC FATIGUE SYNDROME

Chronic Fatigue Immune Dysfunction Syndrome (CFIDS) Association
P.O. Box 220398
Charlotte, NC 28222–0398
800-442-3437
24 hours a day, seven days a week

Provides information and educational materials on the effects of chronic fatigue syndrome. Also supports and funds research.

DENTAL CARE

American Academy of Cosmetic Dentistry
2711 Marshall Ct.
Madison, WI 53705
800-543-9220

Provides information on cosmetic dentistry. Also makes referrals to practitioners in the caller's area.

Environmental Dental Association
9974 Scripps Ranch Blvd., Suite 36
San Diego, CA 92131
800-388-8124

Provides information on alternatives to mercury fillings and how to locate dentists who do not use mercury fillings.

DIABETES MELLITUS

American Diabetes Association
1660 Duke St.
Alexandria, VA 22314
800-232-3472
703-549-1500
8:30 A.M. to 5:00 P.M. (eastern time), Monday to Friday

Provides general information on the diagnosis and treatment of diabetes. Information packet available upon request.

Juvenile Diabetes Foundation
120 Wall St., 19th Floor
New York, NY 10005
800-223-1138
212-889-7575
9:00 A.M. to 5:00 P.M. (eastern time), Monday to Friday
e-mail: Info@jufcure.com

Provides information on the latest research into the causes and prevention of juvenile diabetes. Also provides grants to support ongoing research.

DIGESTIVE DISEASES

Crohn's and Colitis Foundation
444 Park Ave., S
New York, NY 10018
800-343-3637
9:00 A.M. to 5:00 P.M. (eastern time), Monday to Friday

Provides information on digestive diseases and their diagnosis and treatment. Also makes referrals to support groups and chapters in the caller's area. Information packet available upon request.

DISABLED PERSONS' SERVICES

American Paralysis Association
500 Morris Ave.
Springfield, NJ 07081
800-225-0292
800-526-3456 New Jersey
8:30 A.M. to 5:00 P.M. (eastern time), Monday to Friday

Provides information on the treatment of spinal cord injuries. Also makes referrals to support groups in the caller's area. Information packet available upon request.

Architectural and Transportation Barriers Compliance Board
1111 18th St., NW, Suite 501
Washington, DC 20036
800-USA-ABLE (800-872-2253) Voice and TDD
9:00 A.M. to 5:00 P.M. (eastern time), Monday to Friday

Provides information to businesses and other organizations on how to comply with the public accommodations guidelines of the Americans With Disabilities Act as required by Title III.

AT&T National Special Needs Center
2001 Route 46, Suite 310
Parsippany, NJ 07054
800-872-3883
800-833-3232 TDD
8:30 A.M. to 6:30 P.M. (eastern time), Monday to Friday

Provides information on purchasing or renting special equipment and services available to people with hearing, speech, vision or motion impairment.

Devereux Foundation
19 S. Waterloo Rd.
Devon, PA 19333
800-345-1292 Extension 3109
8:45 A.M. to 9:00 P.M. (eastern time), Monday to Friday

Provides information on treatment programs for children, adolescents and adults with psychiatric, emotional, neurological and developmental disabilities. Information packet available upon request.

Equal Employment Opportunity Commission
1801 L St., NW
Washington, DC 20507
800-669-EEOC (800-669-3362)
800-800-3302 TDD
9:00 A.M. to 5:00 P.M. (eastern time), Monday to Friday

Provides information to businesses and other organizations on how to comply with the equal employment opportunity requirements of the Americans With Disabilities Act as required by Title I.

IBM National Support Center for People With Disabilities
P.O. Box 2150
Atlanta, GA 30301
800-426-2133

Provides information on how computers can be used to assist persons with disabilities.

Institute of Logopedics
2400 Jardine Dr.
Wichita, KS 67219
800-835-1043
800-937-4644 Canada
8:00 A.M. to 5:00 P.M. (central time), Monday to Friday

Provides information on residential programs for children with multiple disabilities.

Job Accommodation Network
809 Allen Hall
P.O. Box 6123
West Virginia University
Morgantown, WV 26506–6123
800-526-7234
800-526-4698 West Virginia

Provides information to employers and the public on how to accommodate the needs of persons with disabilities in the workplace.

National Association of Rehabilitation Facilities
P.O. Box 17675
Washington, DC 20041
800-368-3513
8:30 A.M. to 5:30 P.M. (eastern time), Monday to Friday
Answering machine at all other times

Provides the names and locations of rehabilitation facilities. Also makes referrals to support groups in the caller's area.

National Center for Youth With Disabilities
University of Minnesota, Box 721
420 Delaware St., NE
Minneapolis, MN 55455
800-333-6293
612-624-3939 TDD
7:45 A.M. to 4:30 P.M. (central time), Monday to Friday

Provides information to assist parents, educators, caregivers, advocates and others in helping children and youth with disabilities to become fully participating members of society.

National Clearinghouse on Postsecondary Education for Individuals With Disabilities
1 DuPont Circle, Suite 800
Washington, DC 20036–1193
800-544-3284
202-939-9320 District of Columbia

Provides information for individuals with disabilities on job opportunities following graduation from high school.

National Easter Seal Society
230 W. Monroe St., Suite 1800
Chicago, IL 60606–4802
800-221-6827
8:30 A.M. to 5:00 P.M. (central time), Monday to Friday

Provides information on therapy, counseling and educational programs for persons with disabilities. Also makes referrals to community-based programs in the caller's area.

National Information Center for Children and Youth With Disabilities
P.O. Box 1492
Washington, DC 20013
800-695-0285
202-884-8200
9:30 A.M. to 6:30 P.M. (eastern time), Monday to Friday
Answering machine at all other times
e-mail: NICHCY@aed.org

Provides information on programs for children and youth with disabilities.

National Rehabilitation Information Center
8455 Colesville Rd., Suite 935
Silver Spring, MD 20910–3319
800-346-2742
8:00 A.M. to 6:00 P.M. (eastern time), Monday to Friday

Provides information on resources and products for persons with disabilities. Also provides information on research databases that may be used by persons with disabilities.

National Tour Association
Handicapped Travel Division
546 E. Main St.
Lexington, KY 40508
800-682-8886

Provides information to travelers who require special accommodations because of disabilities or other limitations. Provides a list of travel operators who book accommodations for individuals with disabilities.

Pathways Awareness Foundation
123 N. Wacker Dr.
Chicago, IL 60606
800-955-2445
9:00 A.M. to 5:00 P.M. (central time), Monday to Friday

Provides information on the detection of disabilities in early childhood.

Tele-Consumer Hotline
1910 K St., NW, Suite 610
Washington, DC 20006
800-332-1124

Assists persons with disabilities in locating communications equipment that can be adapted to their individual needs.

DOMESTIC VIOLENCE/SEXUAL ABUSE

Hit Home Youth Crisis Line
Youth Development International
P.O. Box 178408
San Diego, CA 92177–8408
800-448-4663
619-292-5683

Provides counseling and referrals on child abuse, runaways, suicide, molestation and pregnancy.

National Child Abuse Hotline
ChildHelp USA
P.O. Box 630
Hollywood, CA 90028
800-422-4453
24 hours a day, seven days a week

Provides crisis counseling and intervention for any abuse-related situation. Also offers information and referral service that includes national, regional or local organizations, agencies and groups. Information packet available upon request.

National Council on Child Abuse and Family Violence
1155 Connecticut Ave., NW, Suite 300
Washington, DC 20036
800-222-2000
202-429-6695 District of Columbia
7:30 A.M. to 4:30 P.M. (eastern time), Monday to Friday

Provides referrals to community services and support groups in the caller's area. Information packet available upon request.

National Resource Center on Child Sexual Abuse
107 Lincoln St.
Huntsville, AL 35801
800-543-7006

Provides resources to agencies dealing with children who have been sexually abused. Also provides bibliographies and articles on the sexual abuse of children.

Parents Anonymous/Abusive Parents
520 S. Lafayette Park Pl., Suite 316
Los Angeles, CA 90057
800-421-0353
800-352-0386 California
8:30 A.M. to 5:00 P.M. (Pacific time), Monday to Friday
Answering machine at all other times

Provides information on the prevention and treatment of child abuse. Also makes referrals to self-help groups and chapters in the caller's area.

DRINKING WATER

GEO/Resource Consultant
1555 Wilson Blvd., Suite 500
Arlington, VA 22209
800-426-4791
8:00 A.M. to 5:00 P.M. (eastern time), Monday to Friday

Provides information on drinking water standards that must be met by community and municipal water suppliers.

DYSLEXIA

Orton Dyslexia Society
Chester Building, Suite 382
8600 LaSalle Rd.
Baltimore, MD 21286–2044
800-222-3123
410-296-0232 Baltimore
9:00 A.M. to 5:00 P.M. (eastern time), Monday to Friday

Provides information on support networks and resources for people with dyslexia.

EATING DISORDERS

Camelback Helpline
7575 E. Earl Dr.
Scottsdale, AZ 85251
800-253-1334
24 hours a day, seven days a week

Provides information on subjects such as mental health, eating disorders and substance dependency. Also makes referrals to treatment centers in the caller's area. Information packet available upon request.

FIT-AHL
Food Addiction Hotline
2000 Commerce St.
Melbourne, FL 32904
800-872-0088
8:00 A.M. to 9:00 P.M. (eastern time), Monday to Friday
9:00 A.M. to 6:00 P.M. (eastern time), Saturday and Sunday

Provides information on eating disorders. Also makes referrals to services in the caller's area. Information packet available upon request.

Take Off Pounds Sensibly (TOPS)
P.O. Box 07630
4575 S. Fifth St.
Milwaukee, WI 53207
800-932-8677
24 hours a day, seven days a week

Provides information on a sensible approach to weight control by showing individuals how to set realistic goals for weight reduction. Also makes referrals to support groups in the caller's area.

EMERGENCY MEDICAL COMMUNICATION SYSTEMS

American Medical Alert Corporation
3265 Lawson Blvd.
Oceanside, NY 11572
800-645-3244

Provides information on telecommunication devices that are used by people with life-threatening conditions or, in the case of accidents, that are used to summon help in emergency situations.

Lifeline Systems
1 Arsenal Marketplace
Watertown, MA 02172
800-451-0525
617-923-4141 Alaska, Hawaii and Massachusetts

Provides information on communication systems that link elderly persons and persons with disabilities directly to hospitals.

ENDOMETRIOSIS

Endometriosis Association
8585 N. 76th Pl.
Milwaukee, WI 53223
800-992-3636
800-426-2363 Canada
24 hours a day, seven days a week

Provides information on the diagnosis and treatment of endometriosis.

Endometriosis Treatment Program
St. Charles Medical Center
2500 N.E. Neff Rd.
Bend, OR 97701
800-446-2177 Extension 6904
541-382-8622
9:00 A.M. to 5:00 P.M. (Pacific time), Monday to Friday

Provides information on the diagnosis and treatment of endometriosis. Offers support and counseling to callers.

ENTERAL/PARENTERAL NUTRITION

Oley Foundation
214 HUN Memorial
Albany Medical Center A-23
Albany, NY 12208
800-776-6539
518-262-5079
9:00 A.M. to 5:00 P.M. (eastern time), Monday to Friday
Answering machine at all other times

Provides information on this specialized system of nutritional therapy to individuals and their families. Publishes a newsletter. Also makes referrals to support groups in the caller's area.

EPILEPSY

Epilepsy Foundation of America
4351 Garden City Dr.
Landover, MD 20785
800-332-1000
9:00 A.M. to 6:00 P.M. (eastern time), Monday to Friday

Provides information on the diagnosis and treatment of epilepsy. Makes referrals to practitioners in the caller's area. Also operates a discount pharmacy available to members.

FACIAL DISFIGUREMENT

About Face USA
P.O. Box 737
Warrington, PA 18976
800-225-3223
24 hours a day, seven days a week

Provides information and support to people with facial disfigurements. Also makes referrals to support groups in the caller's area.

Forward Face
317 E. 34th St., 9th Floor
New York, NY 10016
800-393-3223
212-263-6656
9:00 A.M. to 4:00 P.M. (eastern time), Monday to Friday
Answering machine at all other times

Provides information on craniofacial disorders and support services available. Also maintains links with medical practitioners and publishes a newsletter.

HANSON'S DISEASE

American Leprosy Missions
1 American Leprosy Mission Way
Greenville, SC 29601
800-543-3131
8:00 A.M. to 5:00 P.M. (eastern time), Monday to Friday

Provides information on the diagnosis and treatment of Hanson's disease. Also makes referrals to treatment programs. Information packet available upon request.

HEADACHE

American Council for Headache Education
875 Kings Hwy., Suite 200
West Deptford, NJ 08096
800-255-2243
609-384-8760
24 hours a day, seven days a week

Provides information on the latest research into the causes of headache. Also publishes brochures and patient education materials.

National Headache Foundation
428 W. St. James Pl., 2nd Floor
Chicago, IL 60614
800-843-2256
9:00 A.M. to 5:00 P.M. (central time), Monday to Friday

Provides general information on the diagnosis and treatment of headache. Also makes referrals to support groups in the caller's area.

New England Headache Treatment Program
778 Longridge Rd.
Stamford, CT 06902
800-245-0088
203-968-1799 Connecticut
9:00 A.M. to 4:00 P.M. (eastern time), Monday to Friday

Provides general information on headache and treatment programs available at Greenwich Hospital in Greenwich, Connecticut. Information packet available upon request.

HEAD INJURY

National Head Injury Foundation
1776 Massachusetts Ave., NW, Suite 100
Washington, DC 20036
800-444-6443
202-296-6443 District of Columbia
9:00 A.M. to 5:00 P.M. (eastern time), Monday to Friday

Provides information on the treatment of head injuries. Also makes referrals to support groups in the caller's area.

HEALTH INFORMATION

Agency for Health Care Policy and Research (AHCPR)
U.S. Department of Health and Human Services
AHCPR Publications Clearinghouse
P.O. Box 8547
Silver Spring, MD 20907
800-358-9295
888-586-6340 TDD
410-381-3150
9:00 A.M. to 5:00 P.M. (eastern time), Monday to Friday

Provides information on publications available from the AHCPR dealing with health research studies funded by the federal government. Some publications are available free of charge.

American Institute for Preventive Medicine
30445 Northwestern Hwy.
Farmington Hills, MI 48075
800-345-2476
313-539-1800 Michigan
8:30 A.M. to 5:30 P.M. (eastern time), Monday to Friday

Provides information on programs designed for lifestyle improvement such as stress reduction, weight control, smoking cessation and health education. Information packet available upon request.

American Medical Radio News
515 N. State St.
Chicago, IL 60610
800-448-9384
Provides a recorded message on a current health topic or feature story in medicine.

American Osteopathic Association
142 E. Ontario St.
Chicago, IL 60611
800-621-1773
312-280-5800
8:30 A.M. to 4:30 P.M. (central time), Monday to Friday
Provides information on osteopathic medicine. Also makes referrals to osteopathic physicians and medical centers in the caller's area.

American Trauma Society
8903 Presidential Pkwy., Suite 512
Upper Marlboro, MD 20772–2656
800-556-7890
301-420-4189
9:00 A.M. to 5:00 P.M. (eastern time), Monday to Friday
Provides information on injury prevention and trauma care. Information packet available upon request.

California Self-Help Center
UCLA Psychology Department
405 Hilgard Ave.
Los Angeles, CA 90024
800-222-5465 California
Provides consumer information on a variety of health topics. Also makes referrals to local, regional and national organizations.

Center for Self Help
Riverwood Center
P.O. Box 547
Benton Harbor, MI 49022–0547
800-336-0341 Michigan
Provides information on self-help resources available in the caller's area.

Consumer Health Information Resource Institute
3521 Broadway
Kansas City, MO 64111
800-821-6671
816-753-8850
9:00 A.M. to 5:00 P.M. (central time), Monday to Friday
Provides referrals to local, regional and national organizations. Also maintains a patient education library. Recommends sources of health information on various conditions, procedures and medications.

Doctor Referral Service of Mt. Sinai Medical Center
1 Gustave L. Levy Pl.
P.O. Box 1083
New York, NY 10029–6575
800-637-4624
8:30 A.M. to 6:00 P.M. (eastern time), Monday to Friday

Provides referrals to physicians located in the New York City area who are affiliated with Mt. Sinai Medical Center.

Food and Drug Administration
Office of Consumer Affairs
Parklawn Building
5600 Fishers Ln.
Rockville, MD 20857
800-532-4440
9:00 A.M. to 5:00 P.M. (eastern time), Monday to Friday

Provides information to consumers on Food and Drug Administration actions relative to food and drug items. Also provides consumer education publications and responds to public inquiries.

Health Information Network International
4213 Montgomery Dr.
Santa Rosa, CA 95405
800-743-6996
707-539-3966
9:00 A.M. to 5:00 P.M. (Pacific time), Monday to Friday

Provides consumers with the latest research and information on natural health substances, medical conditions and treatment alternatives.

International Chiropractic Association
1110 N. Glebe Rd.
Arlington, VA 22201
800-423-4690

Provides information on the practice of "straight" chiropractic, which emphasizes spinal manipulation and does not incorporate adjunctive therapies such as heat, cold, ultrasound or vitamins and minerals.

Joseph and Rose Kennedy Institute of Ethics
National Reference Center for Bioethics Literature
Georgetown University
Washington, DC 20057
800-633-3849
202-687-3885

Provides information to medical professionals and the public on medical bioethics.

National Health Information Center
U.S. Department of Health and Human Services
Office of Disease Prevention and Health Promotion
P.O. Box 1133
Washington, DC 20013
800-336-4797
301-565-4167 Maryland
9:00 A.M. to 5:00 P.M. (eastern time), Monday to Friday

Provides information to consumers and professionals on a variety of health-related topics. Also makes referrals to national organizations in the caller's area. Information packet available upon request.

National Institute for Occupational Safety and Health
Department of Health and Human Resources
4676 Columbia Pkwy.
Cincinnati, OH 45226
800-356-4674
24 hours a day, seven days a week

Provides information on workplace safety and compliance with federal occupational and safety regulations.

National Library of Medicine
8600 Rockville Pike, 4th Floor
Bethesda, MD 20894
800-638-8480

Provides information on the services offered at the National Library of Medicine, including computer access to medical literature and information-retrieval systems.

New Jersey Self-Help Clearinghouse
Northwest Covenant Medical Center
25 Pocono Rd.
Denville, NJ 07834–2995
800-367-6274 New Jersey
201-625-7101
201-625-9053 TDD

Provides information to consumers on self-help groups and other organizations. Produces materials on how to establish a self-help group. Also publishes a directory of self-help and mutual-aid organizations.

Office of Minority Health
Resource Center
1010 Wayne Ave., Suite 300
Silver Spring, MD 20910
800-444-6472
9:00 A.M. to 5:00 P.M. (eastern time), Monday to Friday

Provides information to minority groups on health topics that are of special interest to them. Information packet available upon request. English- and Spanish-speaking personnel available to callers.

Office on Smoking and Health Hotline
Centers for Disease Control and Prevention
4770 Buford Hwy., NE, Mailstop K-50
Atlanta, GA 30341–3724
800-CDC-1311 (800-232-1311)
770-488-5705

Provides information on the health effects of smoking and materials relating to smoking-cessation programs.

People's Medical Society
462 Walnut St., Lower Level
Allentown, PA 18102
800-624-8773
8:30 A.M. to 5:00 P.M. (eastern time), Monday to Friday
Answering machine at all other times
e-mail: Peoplesmed@Compuserve.com

Provides information on how to become a better-informed medical consumer. Also publishes consumer-oriented medical information on topics ranging from pediatrics to Medicare. Membership information and publications catalog available upon request.

HEARING IMPAIRMENTS

American Speech-Language-Hearing Association Helpline
10801 Rockville Pike
Rockville, MD 20852
800-638-8255 Voice and TDD
800-897-8682 Alaska, Hawaii and Maryland
301-897-8682
e-mail: IRC@asha.org
8:30 A.M. to 4:30 P.M. (eastern time), Monday to Friday

Provides general information on speech, language and hearing problems. Also makes referrals to practitioners in the caller's area. Information packet available upon request.

Better Hearing Institute
P.O. Box 1840
Washington, DC 20013
800-943-2746
703-642-0580
9:00 A.M. to 5:00 P.M. (eastern time), Monday to Friday
Answering machine at all other times
e-mail: Betterhearing@juno.com

Provides information on deafness and other types of hearing problems.

Captioned Films for the Deaf
5000 Park St., N
St. Petersburg, FL 33709
800-237-6213 Voice and TDD
813-545-8781
8:00 A.M. to 5:00 P.M. (eastern time), Monday to Friday

Provides information on films with captioning that are available for persons with hearing impairments.

Deafness Research Foundation
9 E. 38th St., 7th Floor
New York, NY 10016–0003
800-535-3323 Voice and TTY
212-684-6556 New York City
9:00 A.M. to 5:00 P.M. (eastern time), Monday to Friday

Provides information on hearing problems. Makes referrals to physicians in the caller's area. Also provides information on how to select a hearing aid and detect hearing problems in children. Information packet available upon request.

Delta Society
P.O. Box 1080
Renton, WA 98057–1080
800-869-6898
206-226-7357
9:00 A.M. to 5:00 P.M. (Pacific time), Monday to Friday

Provides information on how to obtain hearing dogs for persons with hearing impairments.

Hear Now
4001 S. Magnolia Way, Suite 100
Denver, CO 80237
800-648-4327 Voice and TDD
303-758-4919 Colorado
8:30 A.M. to 4:00 P.M. (mountain time), Monday to Friday
Answering machine at all other times

Provides information on hearing aids and cochlear implants. Sponsors a national hearing aid bank. Also makes referrals to organizations and agencies in the caller's area.

Hearing Aid Hotline
20361 Middlebelt Rd.
Livonia, MI 48152
800-521-5247
313-478-2610

Provides information on hearing loss and hearing aids. Also makes referrals to hearing aid specialists in the caller's area.

Hearing Information Center
P.O. Box 1880
Media, PA 19063
800-622-3277

Provides hearing screening over the phone and answers general questions about hearing.

National Captioning Institute
5203 Leesburg Pike
Falls Church, VA 22041
800-533-9673
703-998-2443
9:00 A.M. to 5:30 P.M. (eastern time), Monday to Friday
Answering machine at all other times

Provides captioning services for television programs and films. Information packet available upon request.

National Institute on Deafness and Other Communications Disorders
U.S. Department of Health and Human Services
National Institutes of Health Building
9000 Rockville Pike
Bethesda, MD 20892
800-241-1044
800-241-1055 TDD
301-402-0900
8:30 A.M. to 5:30 P.M. (eastern time), Monday to Friday

Provides information on resources that are available to hearing-impaired individuals and their families. Information packet available upon request.

Sensor Hearing Aids
300 S. Chester Rd.
Swarthmore, PA 19081
800-622-3277
215-544-2700
9:00 A.M. to 5:00 P.M. (eastern time), Monday to Friday

Provides information on hearing loss and hearing aids. Also makes referrals to practitioners in the caller's area.

TRIPOD Grapevine
2901 N. Keystone St.
Burbank, CA 91504
800-352-8888 Voice and TDD
800 287-4763 Voice and TDD California
9:00 A.M. to 5:00 P.M. (Pacific time), Monday to Friday

Provides information and services to parents who are raising hearing-impaired children.

HEART DISEASE

American Heart Association
7272 Greenville Ave.
Dallas, TX 75231
800-242-8721
8:30 A.M. to 4:30 P.M. (central time), Monday to Friday

Provides information on coronary conditions. Also makes referrals to support groups in the caller's area.

Coronary Club
9500 Euclid Ave.
Cleveland, OH 44195
800-478-4255
216-444-3690
8:00 A.M. to 4:00 P.M. (eastern time), Monday to Friday
Answering machine at all other times

Provides information on heart care and rehabilitation, including surgery, medication, diet and exercise. Also provides information on the latest research involving the detection and treatment of heart disease.

National Society for MVP and Dysautonomia
880 Montclaire Rd., #280
Birmingham, AL 35213
800-541-8602
205-597-5765
8:15 A.M. to 4:30 P.M. (central time), Monday to Friday

Provides information on the diagnosis and treatment of mitral valve prolapse syndrome and dysautonomia. Also makes referrals to support groups in the caller's area.

HOSPICE

Children's Hospice International
900 N. Washington St., Suite 700
Alexandria, VA 22314
800-242-4453
703-684-0330 Virginia
8:30 A.M. to 5:30 P.M. (eastern time), Monday to Friday
Answering machine at all other times

Provides information on hospice programs especially designed for children with life-threatening conditions or who are terminally ill.

Hospice Education Institute
5 Essex Square
P.O. Box 713
Essex, CT 06246
800-544-2213
203-767-1620 Alaska and Connecticut
9:00 A.M. to 4:30 P.M. (eastern time), Monday to Friday

Provides information and counseling on death and dying and the role of the hospice. Publishes a national directory of hospice programs. Also makes referrals to agencies in the caller's area.

National Hospice Organization
1901 N. Moore St., Suite 901
Arlington, VA 22209
800-658-8898
8:30 A.M. to 5:30 P.M. (eastern time), Monday to Friday

Provides information on hospice programs available in the caller's area.

HOSPITAL CARE

Hill-Burton Hospital Program
Division of Facilities Compliance
Parklawn Building, Room 11-25
5600 Fishers Ln.
Rockville, MD 20857
800-638-0742
800-492-0359 Maryland
9:30 A.M. to 5:30 P.M. (eastern time), Monday to Friday
Answering machine at all other times

Provides information on hospitals that are participating in the Hill-Burton Free Care Program in the caller's area. Information packet available upon request.

HUNTINGTON'S DISEASE

Huntington's Disease Society of America
140 W. 22nd St., 6th Floor
New York, NY 10011–2420
800-345-4372
212-242-1968
9:00 A.M. to 5:00 P.M. (eastern time), Monday to Friday
e-mail: curehd@hdsa.ttisms.com

Provides information and referrals to individuals with Huntington's disease and their families. Also offers crisis intervention and makes referrals to support groups in the caller's area. Information packet available upon request.

IMMUNE DEFICIENCY DISEASES

Immune Deficiency Foundation
Courthouse Square
25 W. Chesapeake Ave., Suite 206
Towson, MD 21204
800-296-4433
9:00 A.M. to 5:00 P.M. (eastern time), Monday to Friday
Answering machine at all other times

Provides information to individuals and families affected by primary immune deficiency diseases. Also publishes educational materials and guidelines on starting support groups in the caller's area.

INCONTINENCE

Help for Incontinent People (HIP)
P.O. Box 544
Union, SC 29379
800-252-3337
803-579-7902
8:00 A.M. to 5:00 P.M. (eastern time), Monday to Friday
Answering machine at all other times

Provides information on incontinence, including latest treatments and developments relating to assistive devices. Also offers suggestions on how to deal with incontinence.

Simon Foundation for Continence
P.O. Box 815
Wilmette, IL 60091
800-237-4666
708-864-3913 Illinois
9:00 A.M. to 6:00 P.M. (central time), seven days a week

Provides information on incontinence. Also makes referrals to practitioners and support groups in the caller's area.

INSURANCE

Alternative Health Insurance Services
P.O. Box 9178
Calabasas, CA 91372–9178
800-331-2713
818-509-5742 Los Angeles

Provides information on insurance plans that cover alternative health-care practitioners.

Communicating for Seniors
P.O. Box 677
Fergus Falls, MN 56538
800-432-3276
218-739-3241
8:00 A.M. to 4:30 P.M. (central time), Monday to Friday

Provides information on insurance matters to older Americans, especially on Medicare supplemental insurance. Information packet available upon request.

Co-op-America
2100 M St., NW, Suite 403
Washington, DC 20037
800-424-2667
202-872-5200 District of Columbia

Provides information on worker-owned and cooperatively structured health insurance plans that provide coverage for conventional as well as alternative practitioners.

National Insurance Consumer Helpline
American Council of Life Insurance
Health Insurance Association of America
Insurance Information Institute
1001 Pennsylvania Ave., NW
Washington, DC 20004
800-942-4242

Provides general information on how to choose an insurance agent or broker and an insurance company. Also provides information on the following types of insurance: health, long-term-care, disability, Medicare supplemental and major medical. Does not provide information on specific policies or companies.

KIDNEY DISEASES

American Association of Kidney Patients
100 S. Ashley Dr., Suite 280
Tampa, FL 33602
800-749-2257
813-251-0725 Tampa
9:00 A.M. to 5:00 P.M. (eastern time), Monday to Friday

Provides information to kidney patients and their families on how to cope with kidney diseases.

American Kidney Fund
6110 Executive Blvd., Suite 1010
Rockville, MD 20852
800-638-8299
800-492-8361 Maryland
8:00 A.M. to 5:00 P.M. (eastern time), Monday to Friday

Provides information on kidney diseases and organ donor programs. Also offers financial assistance to kidney patients. Information packet available upon request.

National Kidney Foundation
30 E. 33rd St.
New York, NY 10016
800-622-9010
8:30 A.M. to 5:30 P.M. (eastern time), Monday to Friday

Provides information on the latest research into kidney and urinary tract diseases, organ donations and transplant programs. Also provides materials for public education programs.

National Medical Care Patient Travel Service
Reservoir Pl.
1601 Trapelo Rd.
Waltham, MA 02154
800-634-6254

Provides information to dialysis patients on how to arrange for dialysis at a National Medical Center dialysis facility while on vacation.

PRK Foundation (polycystic kidney disease)
4901 Main St., Suite 320
Kansas City, MO 64112
800-753-2873
816-931-2600
9:00 A.M. to 5:00 P.M. (central time), Monday to Friday
Answering machine at all other times
e-mail: 75713.2275@Compuserve.com

Provides information on polycystic kidney disease. Also provides support to individuals and their families, raises money for research, publishes a newsletter and sponsors an annual conference.

LEUKODYSTROPHY

United Leukodystrophy Foundation
2304 Highland Dr.
Sycamore, IL 60178
800-728-5483
815-895-3211
24 hours a day, seven days a week
e-mail: ULF@ceet.niu.edu

Provides information on leukodystrophy. Also provides information to caregivers and makes referrals to support groups in the caller's area.

LIVER DISEASES

American Liver Foundation
1425 Pompton Ave.
Cedar Grove, NJ 07009
800-223-0179
201-857-2626 New Jersey
8:30 A.M. to 4:30 P.M. (eastern time), Monday to Friday

Provides information and assistance to children and adults with liver diseases. Also makes referrals to practitioners and support groups in the caller's area.

Wilson's Disease
P.O. Box 75325
Washington, DC 20013
800-399-0266
703-636-3003
24 hours a day, seven days a week

Provides aid and mutual support to individuals and their families affected by Wilson's disease. Promotes research into discovering a treatment and cure for this condition.

LIVING WILLS/ADVANCE DIRECTIVES

Choice in Dying
200 Varick St.
New York, NY 10014
800-989-WILL (800-989-9455)
212-366-5540

Provides information to persons interested in executing living wills or advance directives. Information packet available upon request.

National Hemlock Society
P.O. Box 101810
Denver, CO 80250–1810
800-247-7421

Provides information on the rights of patients to make treatment decisions by executing advance directives.

LUPUS

Lupus Foundation of America
4 Research Pl., Suite 180
Rockville, MD 20850–3226
800-558-0121
301-670-9292 Maryland
24 hours a day, seven days a week

Provides information on books written by doctors and patients who have lupus. Also makes referrals to chapters in the caller's area.

Terri Gothelf Lupus Research Institute
3 Duke Pl.
South Norwalk, CT 06854
800-825-8787
203-852-0120
9:00 A.M. to 7:30 P.M. (eastern time), Monday to Friday

Provides information on medical centers that conduct research into the causes and treatment of lupus. Also provides general information on lupus to patients and their families. Information packet available upon request.

LYME DISEASE

Lyme Disease Foundation
1 Financial Plaza, 18th Floor
Hartford, CT 06103
800-886-LYME (800-866-5963)
860-525-2000
24 hours a day, seven days a week

Provides information on the diagnosis, treatment and prevention of Lyme disease.

LYMPHEDEMA

National Lymphedema Network
2211 Post St., Suite 404
San Francisco, CA 94115–3427
800-541-3259
24 hours a day, seven days a week
e-mail: lymphnet@hooked.net

Provides information on lymphedema to patients and their families. Information packet available upon request.

MARFAN SYNDROME

National Marfan Foundation
382 Main St.
Port Washington, NY 11050
800-862-7326
8:30 A.M. to 3:30 P.M. (eastern time), Monday to Friday
Answering machine at all other times
e-mail: staff@marfan.org

Provides information to individuals who have Marfan syndrome and their families. Also maintains a support network for families, publishes a newsletter and holds conferences.

McCUNE-ALBRIGHT SYNDROME

McCune-Albright Syndrome Division
Magic Foundation
1327 N. Harlem Ave.
Oak Park, IL 60302
800-362-4423
708-383-0808
9:00 A.M. to 5:00 P.M. (central time), Monday to Friday
e-mail: magic@nettap.com

Provides information and support to families of McCune-Albright patients. Also publishes a newsletter with medical information and makes referrals to support groups in the caller's area.

MEDIC ALERT

Medic Alert Foundation International
2323 N. Colorado Ave.
Turlock, CA 95380
800-432-5378
800-468-1020 California
209-668-3333 Alaska and Hawaii
24 hours a day, seven days a week

Provides information on how to register with Medic Alert and obtain an emergency identification bracelet. The foundation also maintains a copy of the patient's medical record, which can be retrieved and sent to a practitioner or medical facility in the event of an emergency. Free registration form and catalog available upon request.

MEDICARE/MEDICAID

Inspector General's Hotline
U.S. Department of Health and Human Services
P.O. Box 17303
Baltimore, MD 21203–7303
800-447-8477
800-638-3986 Maryland
800-269-0271 Social Security issues

Handles complaints from recipients relating to overcharges and possible fraud and waste of funds in the Medicare and Medicaid programs.

Medicare Information Hotline
U.S. Department of Health and Human Services
Health Care Financing Administration
Washington, DC 20201
800-638-6833
8:00 A.M. to midnight, seven days a week

Provides general information on the Medicare program and responds to specific questions concerning Medicare coverage. Also provides information on Medicare supplemental insurance polices. Investigates complaints received from beneficiaries concerning alleged instances of supplemental insurance fraud or abuse.

MEN'S HEALTH

American Prostate Society
1340 Charwood Rd., Suite F
Hanover, MD 21076
800-678-1238
410-850-0818
9:00 A.M. to 5 P.M. (eastern time), Monday to Friday

Provides information on prostate disease and works to increase public awareness. Information packet available upon request.

Impotence Information Center
P.O. Box 9
Minneapolis, MN 55440
800-843-4315
8:00 A.M. to 5:30 P.M. (central time), Monday to Friday
Answering machine at all other times

Provides information on the causes and treatments of impotence but does not provide counseling. Also makes referrals to practitioners in the caller's area.

Star Center
27211 Lahser Rd., Suite 208
Southfield, MI 48034
800-835-7667
313-357-1314 Michigan
24 hours a day, seven days a week

Provides general information on impotency. Also makes referrals to practitioners in the caller's area.

Us Too (Prostate Cancer)
American Foundation for Urologic Disease
300 W. Pratt St., Suite 401
Baltimore, MD 21201
800-828-7866

Provides information on the latest developments in the diagnosis and treatment of prostate cancer. Also makes referrals to chapters in the caller's area.

MÉNIÈRE'S DISEASE

Ménière's Network
Ear Foundation at Baptist Hospital
2000 Church St., Box 111
Nashville, TN 37236
800-545-4327 Extension 304 for TDD
615-329-7807 Voice and TDD
24 hours a day, seven days a week

Provides information on the diagnosis and treatment of Ménière's disease.

MENTAL HEALTH

American Board of Professional Psychology
2100 E. Broadway, Suite 313
Columbia, MO 65201–6082
800-255-7792

Provides information on certified psychologists in the caller's area.

American Mental Health Counselors Association
801 N. Fairfax St., Suite 304
Alexandria, VA 22314
800-326-2642
703-823-9800
8:30 A.M. to 4:30 P.M. (eastern time), Monday to Friday

Provides information on professionals in the counseling field. Also makes referrals to practitioners in the caller's area.

American Mental Health Fund
1021 Price St.
Alexandria, VA 22314
800-433-5959
703-684-2201 Virginia
24 hours a day, seven days a week

Provides general information on mental illness. Also makes referrals to chapters in the caller's area. Information packet available upon request.

American Schizophrenic Association
900 N. Federal Hwy., Suite 330
Boca Raton, FL 33432
800-847-3802
24 hours a day, seven days a week

Provides general information and educational materials about mental illnesses and learning disabilities. Also makes referrals to practitioners in the caller's area. Information packet available upon request.

Camelback Helpline
7575 E. Earl Dr.
Scottsdale, AZ 85251
800-253-1334
24 hours a day, seven days a week

Provides information on subjects such as mental health, eating disorders and substance dependency. Also makes referrals to treatment centers in the caller's area. Information packet available upon request.

Depression/Awareness, Recognition and Treatment Program (D/ART)
National Institute of Mental Health
Inquiries Branch
5600 Fishers Ln.
Rockville, MD 20857
800-421-4211 Spanish available
24 hours a day, seven days a week

Provides information on the causes, treatment and prevention of depression and related mental disorders.

Knowledge Exchange Network (KEN)
National Mental Health Services
P.O. Box 42490
Washington, DC 20001
800-789-2647
301-984-6283
8:30 A.M. to 5:00 P.M. (eastern time), Monday to Friday

Provides information on mental health and resources available to families of those affected by mental health problems. Information packet available upon request.

National Alliance for the Mentally Ill
2101 Wilson Blvd., Suite 302
Arlington, VA 22201
800-950-6264
9:00 A.M. to 5:00 P.M. (eastern time), Monday to Friday
Answering machine at all other times

Provides information on chapters, advocacy and support groups in the caller's area. Information packet available upon request.

National Foundation for Depressive Illness
P.O. Box 2257
New York, NY 10116
800-248-4344
24 hours a day, seven days a week

Provides general information on depression. Also makes referrals to practitioners in the caller's area. Information packet available upon request.

National Mental Health Association
1021 Prince St.
Alexandria, VA 22314–2971
800-969-6642
703-684-7722 Virginia
9:00 A.M. to 6:00 P.M. (eastern time), Monday to Friday

Provides information on mental health and mental illnesses. Also makes referrals to support groups, mental health centers, self-help clearinghouses and other organizations in the caller's area. Information packet available upon request.

MENTAL RETARDATION

American Association on Mental Retardation
444 N. Capital St., NW, Suite 846
Washington, DC 20001–1512
800-424-3688
202-387-1968
9:00 A.M. to 5:00 P.M. (eastern time), Monday to Friday
Answering machine at all other times
e-mail: aamr@access.digex.net

Provides general information on mental retardation. Also makes referrals to practitioners in the caller's area. Information packet available upon request.

MULTIPLE SCLEROSIS

Multiple Sclerosis Association of America
601-05 White Horse Pike
Oaklyn, NJ 08107
800-833-4672
9:00 A.M. to 5:00 P.M. (eastern time), Monday to Friday
Answering machine at all other times

Provides information and support to individuals affected by multiple sclerosis. Publishes a newsletter. Also makes referrals to support groups in the caller's area.

Multiple Sclerosis Foundation
6350 N. Andrew Ave.
Ft. Lauderdale, FL 33309
800-441-7055
305-776-6805
9:00 A.M. to 5:00 P.M. (eastern time), Monday to Friday
e-mail: MSFACTS@icanect.net

Provides information on the latest research into the cause, prevention, treatment and cure of multiple sclerosis. Works to improve the quality of life of people with multiple sclerosis. Also makes referrals to support groups in the caller's area.

MYASTHENIA GRAVIS

Myasthenia Gravis Foundation
53 W. Jackson Blvd., Suite 660
Chicago, IL 60604
800-541-5454
8:00 A.M. to 5:00 P.M. (central time), Monday to Friday

Provides information on the diagnosis and treatment of myasthenia gravis. Also makes referrals to support groups in the caller's area.

NEUROFIBROMATOSIS

Neurofibromatosis
8855 Annapolis Rd., Suite 110
Lanham, MD 20706–2924
800-942-6825
301-577-8984
24 hours a day, seven days a week

Provides information to individuals and families affected by neurofibromatosis. Makes referrals to support groups in the caller's area. Publishes a newsletter and promotes networking among families. Also assists in starting support groups.

NUTRITION INFORMATION

Akpharma Foods
P.O. Box 111
Pleasantville, NJ 08232–0111
800-257-8650
9:00 A.M. to 5:00 P.M. (eastern time), Monday to Friday

Provides information on Beano, a product that helps people digest beans and vegetable fiber. Information packet and samples of the product available upon request.

American Dietetic Association
Consumer Nutrition Hotline
216 W. Jackson Blvd., Suite 800
Chicago, IL 60606
800-366-1655
10:00 A.M. to 5:00 P.M. (central time), Monday to Friday

Provides general information on nutrition, including cholesterol, weight control and healthy snacks. Also makes referrals to nutritional counselors in the caller's area. Provides special service for teenagers.

Beech-Nut Nutrition
Checkerboard Square
Consumer Affairs, 1-B
St. Louis, MO 63164
800-523-6633
800-492-2384 Pennsylvania
9:00 A.M. to 8:00 P.M. (eastern time), Monday to Friday

Provides information on the nutritional content of baby food and answers food-related questions.

Garlic Information Center
Cornell Medical Center
800-330-8922

Provides information on the use of garlic as a seasoning and medicinal product.

Gerber Hotline
Consumer Relations Gerber Products
445 State St.
Fremont, MI 49413
800-443-7237
24 hours a day, seven days a week

Provides information on infant nutrition and specific baby-care topics.

HCF Foundation
High Carbohydrate Fiber
University of Kentucky
800 Rose St.
Lexington, KY 40536
800-727-4423

Provides information on the role of dietary fiber in regard to cholesterol, diabetes and blood sugar levels. Callers may leave specific questions on the voice-mail system.

International Olive Oil Council
P.O. Box 2506
Stuart, FL 34995–2506
800-232-6548
9:00 A.M. to 5:00 P.M. (eastern time), Monday to Friday

Provides information on the nutritional and fat content of olive oil. Information packet available upon request.

Lactaid
McNeil Consumer Affairs
P.O. Box 85
Camp Hill Road
Ft. Washington, PA 19034
800-522-8243
9:00 A.M. to 5:00 P.M. (eastern time), Monday to Friday

Provides information on lactose intolerance and Lactaid, a product that assists in the digestion of lactose. Information packet and samples available upon request.

Meat and Poultry Hotline
U.S. Department of Agriculture
Room 1165 S, FSIS
Washington, DC 20250
800-535-4555
202-720-3333 District of Columbia
10:00 A.M. to 4:00 P.M. (eastern time), Monday to Friday

Provides information on the proper handling and storage of meat and poultry products. Information packet available upon request.

Molly McButter Information Hotline
800-622-3274
9:00 A.M. to 5:00 P.M. (eastern time), Monday to Friday

Provides information on the fat and calorie content of foods. Callers may speak directly with registered dietitians.

Mrs. Dash Sodium Information Hotline
800-622-3274
9:00 A.M. to 5:00 P.M. (eastern time), Monday to Friday

Provides low-sodium recipes and information on the sodium content of foods for people on sodium-restricted diets. Information packet available upon request.

Nutrition Hotline
American Institute for Cancer Research
1759 R St., NW
Washington, DC 20009
800-843-8114
202-328-7744 District of Columbia
9:00 A.M. to 9:00 P.M. (eastern time), Monday to Thursday
9:00 A.M. to 5:00 P.M. (eastern time), Friday
Answering machine at all other times

Provides information on the role of diet and nutrition in cancer prevention and how nutrition may be used to assist a cancer treatment program. Also responds to specific requests for information.

Seafood Hotline
U.S. Department of Health and Human Services
Food and Drug Administration
Rockville, MD 20857
800-FDA-4010 (800-332-4010)
202-205-4314 District of Columbia
10:00 A.M. to 2:00 P.M. (eastern time), Monday to Friday
Answering machine at all other times

Provides information on how to buy and use seafood products. Callers may speak directly to food specialists or access prerecorded information on the proper handling and storage of seafood. List of seafood publications from the Food and Drug Administration available upon request.

ORGAN DONOR PROGRAMS

The Living Bank
P.O. Box 6725
Houston, TX 77265
800-528-2971
713-528-2971
24 hours a day, seven days a week

Operates a registry and referral program for people wishing to donate their vital organs or bodies to research.

National Marrow Donor Program
3433 Broadway St., NE, Suite 400
Minneapolis, MN 55413–1762
800-654-1247 Extension 149 for Spanish
8:00 A.M. to 6:00 P.M. (central time), Monday to Friday
Answering machine at all other times

Provides information on how to become a bone marrow donor.

Organ Donor Hotline
United Network for Organ Sharing
1100 Boulders Pkwy., Suite 500
P.O. Box 13770
Richmond, VA 23225–8770
800-355-7527
804-330-8602
9:00 A.M. to 5:00 P.M. (eastern time), Monday to Friday
Answering machine at all other times

Provides information on organ donor programs and transplants. Also provides organ donor cards upon request.

Transplant Recipients International Organization (TRIO)
1000 16th St., NW, Suite 602
Washington, DC 20036–5705
800-874-6386
9:00 A.M. to 5:00 P.M. (eastern time), Monday to Friday
Answering machine at all other times
e-mail: trio@primenet.com

Provides information and peer support to transplant recipients and their families. Conducts public education programs on the importance of organ donation. Also makes referrals to chapters in the caller's area.

ORPHAN DRUGS AND RARE DISEASES

Friends of Karen
P.O. Box 190
Purdys, NY 10578
800-637-2774
9:00 A.M. to 5:00 P.M. (eastern time), Monday to Friday

Provides information on financial support that may be available to families with children who have rare or life-threatening diseases. Also provides information on support groups. Information packet available upon request.

National Information Center for Orphan Drugs and Rare Diseases
P.O. Box 1133
Washington, DC 20013
800-336-4797
202-429-9091 District of Columbia
9:00 A.M. to 5:00 P.M. (eastern time), Monday to Friday
e-mail: nhicinfo@health.org

Provides information on how to locate a source for orphan drugs. (Orphan drugs, for which there is only a small market, are used to treat rare illnesses.)

National Information Clearinghouse for Infants With Disabilities and Life-Threatening Conditions
University of South Carolina
Benson Building, 1st Floor
Columbia, SC 29208
800-922-9234 Voice and TDD
800-922-1107 Voice and TDD South Carolina
9:00 A.M. to 5:00 P.M. (eastern time), Monday to Friday
Answering machine at all other times

Provides information to families with children who have rare or life-threatening conditions. Also makes referrals to professional and community services in the caller's area. Offers special services to Vietnam veterans and their families.

National Organization for Rare Disorders
P.O. Box 8923
New Fairfield, CT 06812–1783
800-447-6673
800-833-8134 TDD
9:00 A.M. to 5:00 P.M. (eastern time), Monday to Friday
Answering machine at all other times

Provides information on how to apply for the drug cost-sharing program sponsored by the pharmaceutical industry. Information packet available upon request.

OSTEOPOROSIS

National Osteoporosis Foundation
1150 17th St., NW, Suite 500
Washington, DC 20036–4603
800-223-9994
202-223-2226

Provides information on osteoporosis, including a publication answering basic questions about the condition. Information packet available upon request.

OSTOMY

United Ostomy Association
36 Executive Park, #120
Irvine, CA 92714–6744
800-826-0826
714-660-8624
7:00 A.M. to 4:00 P.M. (Pacific time), Monday to Friday
Answering machine at all other times

Provides information on ostomy procedures and helps those with ostomies to lead normal lives. Also makes referrals to support groups in the caller's area. Information packet available upon request.

OVER-THE-COUNTER MEDICATIONS

The following manufacturers of over-the-counter medications may be contacted for more information on the proper use of their products. Information lines are available 24 hours a day unless otherwise indicated.

3M Personal Health Care
Building 515-3N-02
St. Paul, MN 55144–1000
800-537-2191

American Lifeline
103 S. Second St.
Madison, WI 53704
800-257-5433

AML Laboratories
1753 Cloverfield Blvd.
Santa Monica, CA 90404
800-800-1200

Astra USA
50 Otis St.
Westborough, MA 01581–4500
800-262-0460

Bausch & Lomb
Personal Products Division
1400 N. Goodman St.
P.O. Box 450
Rochester, NY 14692–0450
800-553-5340

Bayer Corporation
Consumer Care Division
36 Columbia Rd.
Morristown, NJ 07960–4518
800-331-4536

Blaine Company
1465 Jamike Ln.
Erlanger, KY 41018
800-633-9353

Blairex Laboratories
3240 N. Indianapolis Rd.
P.O. Box 2127
Columbus, IN 47202–2127
800-252-4739

Boiron
6 Campus Blvd., Building A
Newtown Square, PA 19073
800-258-8823

Bristol-Myers Products
345 Park Ave.
New York, NY 10154
800-468-7746

Care-Tech Laboratories
3224 S. Kingshighway Blvd.
St. Louis, MO 63139
800-325-9681

Church & Dwight Company
469 N. Harrison St.
Princeton, NJ 08543–5297
800-228-5635

Efcon Laboratories
P.O. Box 7499
Marietta, GA 30065–1499
800-722-2428

Iyata Pharmaceutical
735 N. Water St., Suite 612
Milwaukee, WI 53202
800-809-7918

Kyolic
Division of Wakunaga of America Company
23501 Madero St.
Mission Viejo, CA 92691
800-421-2998

Lederle Consumer Health
A Division of Whitehall-Robins Healthcare
5 Giralda Farms
Madison, NJ 07940–0821
800-282-8805

Marlyn Nutraceuticals
14851 N. Scottsdale Rd.
Scottsdale, AZ 85254
800-462-7596

McNeil Consumer Products
Division of McNeil-PPC
1 Campus Dr.
Somerset, NJ 08873
800-523-6225

Muro Pharmaceutical
890 East St.
Tewksbury, MA 01876–1496
800-225-0974

Ohm Laboratories
P.O. Box 7397
North Brunswick, NJ 08902
800-527-6481

Pfizer Pharmaceuticals
Consumer Health Care Group
Division of Pfizer
235 E. 42nd St.
New York, NY 10017–5755
800-723-7529

Pharmaton Natural Health Products
A Division of Boehringer Ingelheim Pharmaceutical
900 Ridgebury Rd.
Ridgefield, CT 06877
800-243-0127

Procter & Gamble
P.O. Box 5516
Cincinnati, OH 45201
800-358-8707

Requa
P.O. Box 4008
1 Senneca Pl.
Greenwich, CT 06830
800-321-1085

Roberts Pharmaceutical Corporation
4 Industrial Way, W
Eatontown, NJ 07724
800-828-2088

Ross Products Division
Abbott Laboratories
Columbus, OH 43215–1724
800-227-5767

Similasan Corporation
1321 S. Central Ave.
Kent, WA 98032
800-426-1644

SmithKline Beecham Consumer Healthcare
Unit of SmithKline Beecham
P.O. Box 1467
Pittsburgh, PA 15230
800-245-1040

Stellar Pharmacal Corporation
1990 N.W. 44th St.
Pompano Beach, FL 33064–8712
800-845-7827

Triton Consumer Products
561 E. Golf Rd.
Arlington Heights, IL 60005
800-942-2009

Wallace Laboratories
P.O. Box 1001
Half Acre Road
Cranbury, NJ 08512
800-526-3840

Warner-Lambert Consumer Helpline
Warner-Lambert Company
Consumer Health Products Group
201 Tabor Rd.
Morris Plains, NJ 07950
800-524-2854
800-223-0182

Whitehall-Robins Healthcare
American Home Products Corporation
5 Giralda Farms
Madison, NJ 07940–0871
800-322-3129
800-762-4672

PARALYSIS AND SPINAL CORD INJURY

APA Spinal Cord Injury Hotline
2200 Kernane Dr.
Baltimore, MD 21207
800-526-3456
9:00 A.M. to 5:00 P.M. (eastern time), Monday to Friday
Answering machine at all other times
e-mail: SCIHOTLINE@aol.com

Provides information on spinal cord injuries. Also makes referrals to organizations, agencies and treatment centers in the caller's area.

American Paralysis Association
Montebello Hospital
500 Morris Ave.
Springfield, NJ 07081
800-225-0292
201-379-2690 New Jersey
9:00 A.M. to 5:00 P.M. (eastern time), Monday to Friday
e-mail: Paralysis@aol.com

Provides information on the latest research into the treatment of spinal cord injuries and prospects for recovery. Information packet available upon request.

National Spinal Cord Injury Association
8300 Colesville Rd., Suite 551
Silver Spring, MD 20910
800-962-9629
9:00 A.M. to 5:00 P.M. (eastern time), Monday to Friday
e-mail: NSCI2@aol.com

Provides information to patients and their families on services available from organizations, agencies and support groups in the caller's area. Information packet available upon request.

PARENTING

A Way Out
P.O. Box 277
New Paltz, NY 12561
800-292-9688
914-255-1907
24 hours a day, seven days a week

Provides assistance to parents who are considering abducting their children or who already have taken their children. Also has a network of nationwide mediators who can help resolve custody disputes between parents.

Child Reach
155 Plan Way
Warwick, RI 02886
800-556-7918 Extension 216 for TDD

Provides information on how to become a sponsor to a child living in the Third World.

National Association for Parents of the Visually Impaired
P.O. Box 317
Watertown, MA 02272–0317
800-562-6265
617-924-3434
9:00 A.M. to 5:00 P.M. (eastern time), Monday to Friday

Provides general information and counseling to families with visually impaired children.

Parents Without Partners
8807 Colesville Rd.
Silver Spring, MD 20910
800-637-7974
301-588-9354 Maryland
9:00 A.M. to 5:00 P.M. (central time), Monday to Friday

Provides information on support groups for single parents. Information packet available upon request.

Technical Assistance to Parent Programs Network
Federation for Children With Special Needs
95 Berkeley St., Suite 104
Boston, MA 02116
800-331-0688 Massachusetts
9:00 A.M. to 5:00 P.M. (eastern time), Monday to Friday

Provides information to parents with children who have special needs because of developmental disabilities, including information on special education laws. Offers training and workshops for parents of children with special needs. Also makes referrals to support groups in the caller's area.

Toughlove International
P.O. Box 1069
Doylestown, PA 18901
800-333-1069
215-348-7090 Pennsylvania

Serves as a support group for parents of teenage children with behavioral problems. Also makes referrals in both the United States and Canada.

PARKINSON'S DISEASE

American Parkinson's Disease Association
1250 Hylan Blvd.
Staten Island, NY 10305
800-223-2732 New York
719-981-8001
9:00 A.M. to 5:00 P.M. (eastern time), Monday to Friday
Answering machine at all other times

Provides brochures and information packets on medicines used to treat Parkinson's disease. Also offers counseling services and makes referrals to treatment centers in the caller's area.

National Parkinson's Foundation
1501 N.W. Ninth Ave.
Miami, FL 33136
800-327-4545
800-433-7022 Florida
305-547-6666 Miami
8:00 A.M. to 5:00 P.M. (eastern time), Monday to Friday
e-mail: mailbox@NPF.Med.miami.edu

Provides information on Parkinson's disease. Also makes referrals to practitioners in the caller's area.

Parkinson's Disease Foundation
William Black Medical Research Building
710 W. 168th St.
New York, NY 10032
800-457-6676
9:00 A.M. to 5:00 P.M. (eastern time), Monday to Friday
e-mail: PDFCPMC@aol.com

Provides information on patient care and rehabilitation, including lists of self-help groups and of clinics where treatment is available. Clinical specialists are available to answer questions from callers.

PESTICIDES

National Pesticides Telecommunications Network
National Pesticides Information Clearinghouse
Oregon State University
333 Weniger Hall
Corvalis, OR 97332–6502
800-858-7378
541-737-1197 TDD
24 hours a day, seven days a week
e-mail: MILLERT@ACE.ORST.EDU

Provides information to the public and the medical profession on the hazards of pesticides.

PHARMACEUTICAL MANUFACTURERS
(Free Medication Program)

The following companies provide free medicine for economically disadvantaged persons through patient-assistance programs. Most of these companies ask that patients meet certain income requirements. Check with the individual companies to learn the requirements and the process for submitting an application.

Abbott Laboratories/Ross Laboratories
1 Abbott Park Rd.
Abbott Park, IL 60064–3500
800-922-3255
708-937-6100

Allergan Prescription Pharmaceuticals
2525 Dupont Dr.
P.O. Box 19534
Irvine, CA 92713–9534
800-347-4500 Extension 6219
714-752-4500

Amgen
1840 Deharilland Dr.
Thousand Oaks, CA 91320–1789
800-272-9376
805-447-1000

Bristol-Myers Squibb
Bristol-Myers U.S. Pharmaceutical Division
P.O. Box 4500
Princeton, NJ 08543–4500
800-736-0003
609-897-2000

Genentech
460 Point San Bruno Blvd.
South San Francisco, CA 94080
800-879-4747
415-225-1000

GlaxoWellcome
5 Moore Dr.
P.O. Box 13408
Research Triangle Park, NC 27709
800-452-9677
919-248-2100

Hoechst-Marion-Roussel
Routes 202-206
P.O. Box 2500
Somerville, NJ 08876–1258
800-776-4563
908-231-2000

Hoffman-La Roche
340 Kingsland St.
Nutley, NJ 07110
800-526-6367
201-235-5000

Pfizer Pharmaceuticals
235 E. 42nd St.
New York, NY 10017–5755
800-869-9979
212-573-2323

Sandoz Pharmaceuticals Corporation
59 Route 10
East Hanover, NJ 07936
800-937-6673
201-503-7500

PHYSICIAN CREDENTIALING

ABMS Certification Line
American Board of Medical Specialties
47 Perimeter Center, E, Suite 500
Atlanta, GA 30346
800-776-2378
9:00 A.M. to 6:00 P.M. (eastern time), Monday to Friday

Provides information on the certification status of physicians, including their specialties and years in which they were certified. Caller should have physician's name and location ready before calling.

American Osteopathic Association
Department of Certification
142 E. Ontario St.
Chicago, IL 60611
800-621-1773
312-280-5845
9:00 A.M. to 5:00 P.M. (central time), Monday to Friday

Provides information on osteopathy as a healing art. Also verifies the specialty board certification of osteopathic physicians.

POISON CONTROL CENTERS

See also: **PESTICIDES** and **TOXIC SUBSTANCES**

Note: *The following poison control centers are certified by the* ***American Association of Poison Control Centers (AAPCC),*** *3201 New Mexico Ave., NW, Suite 310, Washington, DC 20016. There may be other poison control centers in your area; however, these are the only centers that meet AAPCC standards. Unless otherwise indicated, the toll-free number is only available in the state, section of the state or area code shown.* ***In the event of an emergency, contact the nearest hospital serving your area.***

ALABAMA

Alabama Poison Center
408-A Paul Bryant Dr.
Tuscaloosa, AL 35401
800-462-0800
205-345-0600 Tuscaloosa

Regional Poison Center
Children's Hospital of Alabama
1600 Seventh Ave., S
Birmingham, AL 35233
800-292-6678
205-939-9201 Birmingham
205-933-4050 Birmingham

ARIZONA

Arizona Poison and Drug Information Center
University of Arizona
Arizona Health Science Center, Room 1156
1501 N. Campbell Ave.
Tucson, AZ 85724
800-362-0101
520-626-6016 Tucson

Samaritan Regional Poison Center
Good Samaritan Regional Medical Center
Ancillary-1
1111 E. McDowell Rd.
Phoenix, AZ 85006
602-253-3334 Phoenix

CALIFORNIA

Central California Regional Poison Control Center
Valley Children's Hospital
3151 N. Millbrook, IN31
Fresno, CA 93703
800-346-5922 Central California
209-445-1222 Fresno

Regional Poison Control Center
University of California-Davis Medical Center
2315 Stockton Blvd.
Sacramento, CA 95817
800-342-9293 Northern California
916-734-3692 Sacramento

San Diego Regional Poison Center
University of California San Diego Medical Center
200 W. Arbor Dr.
San Diego, CA 92103–8925
800-876-4766 Accessible in area code 619

COLORADO

Rocky Mountain Poison and Drug Center
8802 E. Ninth Ave.
Denver, CO 80220
800-332-3073 Colorado
303-629-1123 Denver
800-860-0620 Idaho
800-525-5042 Montana
800-446-6179 Las Vegas

CONNECTICUT

Connecticut Poison Control Center
University of Connecticut Health Center
263 Farmington Ave.
Farmington, CT 06030
800-343-2722
203-679-3056 Farmington

DISTRICT OF COLUMBIA

National Capitol Poison Center
3201 New Mexico Ave., NW, Suite 310
Washington, DC 20016
202-625-3333
202-362-8563 TTY

FLORIDA

Florida Poison Information Center-Jacksonville
University Medical Center
University of Florida Health Science Center-Jacksonville
655 W. Eighth St.
Jacksonville, FL 32009
800-282-3171
904-549-4480 Jacksonville

Florida Poison Information Center-Miami
University of Miami School of Medicine
Department of Pediatrics
P.O. Box 016960 (R-131)
Miami, FL 33101
800-282-3171

Florida Poison Information Center and Toxicology Resource Center
Tampa General Hospital
P.O. Box 1289
Tampa, FL 33601
800-282-3171
813-253-4444 Tampa

GEORGIA

Georgia Regional Poison Control Center
Grady Memorial Hospital
80 Butler St., SE
P.O. Box 26066
Atlanta, GA 30335
800-282-5846
404-616-9000 Atlanta

INDIANA

Indiana Poison Control Center
Methodist Hospital of Indiana
1701 N. Senate Blvd.
P.O. Box 1367
Indianapolis, IN 46206
800-382-9097 Northern Indiana, northern Ohio, central and southern Michigan
317-929-2323 Indianapolis

KENTUCKY

Kentucky Regional Poison Center
Kosair Children's Hospital
Medical Towers South, Suite 572
P.O. Box 35070
Louisville, KY 40232
800-722-5725
502-589-8222 Louisville and southern Indiana

LOUISIANA

Louisiana Drug and Poison Information Center
Northeast Louisiana University
Sugar Hall
Monroe, LA 71209
800-256-9822
318-362-5393 Monroe

MARYLAND

Maryland Poison Center
University of Maryland School of Pharmacy
20 N. Pine St.
Baltimore, MD 21201
800-492-2414 Maryland
410-528-7701 Baltimore

National Capitol Poison Center (DC suburbs only)
3201 New Mexico Ave., NW, Suite 310
Washington, DC 20016
202-625-3333
202-362-8563 TTY

MASSACHUSETTS

Massachusetts Poison Control System
300 Longwood Ave.
Boston, MA 02115
800-682-9211
617-232-2120 Boston

MICHIGAN

Poison Control Center
Children's Hospital of Michigan
Harper Professional Building
4160 John Rd., Suite 425
Detroit, MI 48201
313-745-5711 Detroit

MINNESOTA

Hennepin Regional Poison Center
Hennepin County Medical Center
701 Park Ave.
Minneapolis, MN 55415
612-347-3141 Minneapolis
612-337-7474 TDD
612-337-7387 Petline

Minnesota Regional Poison Center
8100 34th Ave., S
P.O. Box 1309
Minneapolis, MN 55440–1309
612-221-2113 Minneapolis

MISSOURI

Regional Poison Center
Cardinal Glennon Children's Hospital
1465 S. Grand Blvd.
St. Louis, MO 63104
800-366-8888 Also serves western Illinois, Missouri and Topeka, Kansas
314-772-5200 St. Louis

MONTANA

Rocky Mountain Poison and Drug Center
8802 E. Ninth Ave.
Denver, CO 80220
800-525-5042 Montana

NEBRASKA

The Poison Center
Children's Memorial Hospital
8301 Dodge St.
Omaha, NE 68114
800-955-9119 Nebraska and Wyoming
402-390-5555 Omaha

NEW JERSEY

New Jersey Poison Information and Education System
Newark Beth Israel Medical Center
201 Lyons Ave.
Newark, NJ 07112
800-962-1253

NEW MEXICO

New Mexico Poison and Drug Information Center
University of New Mexico, North Campus
Health Science Library, Room 125
Albuquerque, NM 87131
800-432-6866
505-843-2551 Albuquerque

NEW YORK

Central New York Poison Control Center
SUNY Health Science Center
750 E. Adams St.
Syracuse, NY 13203
800-252-5655
315-476-4766 Syracuse

Finger Lakes Regional Poison Center
University of Rochester Medical Center
601 Elmwood Ave.
Box 321, Room G-3275
Rochester, NY 14642
800-333-0542
716-275-5151 Rochester

Hudson Valley Regional Poison Center
Phelps Memorial Hospital Center
701 N. Broadway
North Tarrytown, NY 10591
800-336-6997
914-366-3030 North Tarrytown

Long Island Regional Poison Control Center
Winthrop University Hospital
259 First St.
Mineola, NY 11501
516-542-2323 Mineola
516-542-2324 Mineola
516-542-2325 Mineola
516-542-3813 Mineola

New York City Poison Control Center
New York City Department of Health
455 First Ave., Room 123
New York, NY 10016
212-340-4494
212-689-9014 TDD

NORTH CAROLINA

Carolinas Poison Center
1012 S. Kings Dr., Suite 206
P.O. Box 32861
Charlotte, NC 28232
800-848-6946
704-355-4000 Charlotte

NORTH DAKOTA

North Dakota Poison Information Center
MediCare Medical Center
720 Fourth St., N
Fargo, ND 58122
800-732-2200
701-234-5575 Fargo

OHIO

Central Ohio Poison Control Center
Children's Hospital
700 Children's Dr.
Columbus, OH 43205
800-682-7625
614-228-2272 TTY
614-228-1323 Columbus

Cincinnati Drug and Poison Information Center and Regional Poison Control Systems
P.O. Box 670144
Cincinnati, OH 45267
800-872-5111
513-558-5111 Cincinnati

OREGON

Oregon Poison Center
Oregon Health Sciences University
3181 S.W. Sam Jackson Park Rd., CB550
Portland, OR 97201
800-452-7165
503-494-8968 Portland

PENNSYLVANIA

Central Pennsylvania Poison Center
University Hospital
Milton S. Hershey Medical Center
University Drive
P.O. Box 850
Hershey, PA 17033
800-521-6110
717-531-8335 TDD

Pittsburgh Poison Center
3705 Fifth Ave.
Pittsburgh, PA 15213
412-681-6669 Pittsburgh

The Poison Control Center
3600 Sciences Center, Suite 220
Philadelphia, PA 19104
800-521-6110
215-386-2100 Philadelphia

RHODE ISLAND

Rhode Island Poison Center
593 Eddy St.
Providence, RI 02903
401-444-5727 Providence

TENNESSEE

Middle Tennessee Poison Center
The Center for Clinical Toxicology
Vanderbilt University Medical Center
1161 21st Ave., S
501 Oxford House
Nashville, TN 37232
800-288-9999 Accessible in area code 615

TEXAS

Central Texas Poison Center
Scott & White Memorial Hospital
2401 S. 31st St.
Temple, TX 76508
800-764-7661

North Texas Poison Center
Parkland Hospital
5201 Harry Hines Blvd.
P.O. Box 35926
Dallas, TX 75235
800-441-0040
800-764-7661

Southeast Texas Poison Center
University of Texas Medical Branch
301 University Ave.
Galveston, TX 77550
800-764-7661
409-765-1420 Galveston
713-654-1701 Houston

UTAH

Utah Poison Control Center
410 Chipeta Way, Suite 230
Salt Lake City, UT 84108
800-456-7707 Utah
801-581-2151 Salt Lake City

VIRGINIA

Blue Ridge Poison Center
Box 67, Blue Ridge
University of Virginia Medical Center
Charlottesville, VA 22901
800-451-1428 Central, northern and western Virginia
804-924-5543 Charlottesville

National Capitol Poison Center (northern Virginia only)
3201 New Mexico Ave., NW, Suite 310
Washington, DC 20016
202-625-3333
202-362-8563 TTY

WASHINGTON

Washington Poison Center
155 N.E. 100th St., Suite 400
Seattle, WA 98125
800-732-6985
800-572-0638 TDD
206-526-2121 Seattle
206-517-2394 Seattle

WEST VIRGINIA

West Virginia Poison Center
West Virginia University School of Pharmacy
3110 MacCorkle Ave., SE
Charleston, WV 25304
800-642-3625
304-348-4211 Charleston

WYOMING

The Poison Center
Children's Memorial Hospital
8301 Dodge St.
Omaha, NE 68114
800-955-9119 Nebraska and Wyoming

PREGNANCY SERVICES

Abortion Hotline
National Abortion Federation
1436 U St., NW
Washington, DC 20009
800-772-9100
202-667-5881 District of Columbia
9:30 A.M. to 5:30 P.M. (eastern time), Monday to Friday

Provides information on services available at clinics in the caller's area. Also provides information on state laws applicable to abortion services.

American Academy of Husband-Coached Childbirth
P.O. Box 5224
Sherman Oaks, CA 91413–5224
800-422-4784
818-788-6662 Sherman Oaks
24 hours a day, seven days a week

Provides information on the Bradley method of childbirth. Also makes referrals to practitioners in the caller's area. Information packet, including a directory of instructors, available upon request.

American Society for Psychoprophylaxis in Obstetrics/Lamaze
1200 19th St., NW, Suite 300
Washington, DC 20036
800-368-4404
202-857-1128 District of Columbia
9:00 A.M. to 5:00 P.M. (eastern time), Monday to Friday
e-mail: aspo@sba.com

Provides information on the Lamaze technique. Also makes referrals to chapters in the caller's area.

Be Healthy: Positive Pregnancy and Parenting Fitness
51 Saltrock Rd.
Baltic, CT 06330
800-433-5523
203-822-8573 Connecticut
9:00 A.M. to 5:00 P.M. (eastern time), Monday to Friday
Answering machine at all other times

Provides information on pregnancy and parenting, including audio and visual aids. Information packet available upon request.

Bethany Christian Services
901 Eastern Ave., NE
Grand Rapids, MI 49503
800-238-4269
8:00 A.M. to midnight (eastern time), Monday to Friday
e-mail: LL@Bethany.org

Provides pregnancy testing, counseling services and adoption services to women. Information packet available upon request.

Birthright
686 N. Broad St.
Woodbury, NJ 08096
800-848-5683
609-848-1818 New Jersey
8:00 A.M. to 3:00 P.M. (eastern time), Monday to Friday

Provides confidential pregnancy counseling to adolescents and women who are homeless because of their pregnancy. Also provides maternity and baby clothes and support services such as medical and financial referrals.

Depression After Delivery
P.O. Box 1282
Morrisville, PA 19067
800-944-4774
215-295-3994
24 hours a day, seven days a week

Provides information to women who are experiencing postpartum depression. Also makes referrals to telephone support networks in the caller's area. Guidelines for starting support groups available upon request.

Edna Gladney Center Pregnancy Hotline
2300 Hemphill St.
Ft. Worth, TX 76110
800-452-3639
817-926-3304 Texas
8:00 A.M. to 9:00 P.M. (central time), Monday to Friday

Provides information on all the options of pregnancy, especially adoption. Provides residential services to women who are considering placing their babies for adoption.

Emergency Contraception Hotline
American College of Obstetricians and Gynecologists
409 12th St., SW
P.O. Box 96920
Washington, DC 20090–6920
800-584-9911
202-638-5577

Provides information and counseling on the steps to be taken to prevent conception in an emergency situation.

International Childbirth Education Association
P.O. Box 20048
Minneapolis, MN 55420
800-624-4934

Provides information on pregnancy, childbirth and other related infant health needs. Also operates a book center. Information packet and catalog available upon request.

La Leche League International
P.O. Box 1209
9616 Minneapolis Ave.
Franklin Park, IL 60131–8209
800-525-3243
9:00 A.M. to 3:00 P.M. (central time), Monday to Friday

Provides information on breast-feeding.

Planned Parenthood Federation of America
810 Seventh Ave.
New York, NY 10019
800-829-7732
8:30 A.M. to 5:00 P.M. (eastern time), Monday to Friday

Provides information on family planning matters, including the use of contraceptives. Also makes referrals to Planned Parenthood clinics in the caller's area.

PREMENSTRUAL SYNDROME (PMS)

PMS Access
P.O. Box 9326
Madison, WI 53715
800-222-4767
608-257-8682 Wisconsin
9:00 A.M. to 5:00 P.M. (central time), Monday to Friday
Answering machine at all other times

Provides information on all aspects of premenstrual syndrome. Also makes referrals to practitioners in the caller's area. Information packet available upon request.

PRODUCT SAFETY

U.S. Consumer Product Safety Commission
5401 Westbard Ave.
Bethesda, MD 20207
800-638-CPSC (800-638-3772)
800-638-8270 TDD
800-492-8104 TDD Maryland
9:00 A.M. to 5:00 P.M. (eastern time), Monday to Friday

Provides information on how to report complaints of injuries caused by consumer products.

PSEUDOTUMOR CEREBRI

Pseudotumor Cerebri Society
1319 Butternut St., #3
Syracuse, NY 13208
800-926-1230
9:00 A.M. to 5:00 P.M. (eastern time), Monday to Friday

Provides information on the diagnosis and treatment of this condition. Also makes referrals to support groups in the caller's area.

RETINITIS PIGMENTOSA

National Retinitis Pigmentosa Foundation
Executive Plaza One, Suite 800
11350 McCormick Rd.
Hunt Valley, MD 21031–1014
800-683-5555
800-683-5551 TDD
410-225-9400 Maryland
8:30 A.M. to 5:00 P.M. (eastern time), Monday to Friday
Answering machine at all other times

Provides information on the latest developments in the treatment of retinitis pigmentosa and responds to questions from callers.

Retinitis Pigmentosa International Fighting Blindness
P.O. Box 900
Woodland Hills, CA 91365
800-344-4877
24 hours a day, seven days a week

Provides information on retinitis pigmentosa and reports on the latest research into the diagnosis and treatment of this condition.

REYE'S SYNDROME

National Reye's Syndrome Foundation
426 N. Lewis St.
P.O. Box 8292
Bryan, OH 43506
800-233-7393
800-231-7393 Ohio
24 hours a day, seven days a week
e-mail: REYESSYN@mail.bright.net

Provides information on the symptoms and treatment of Reye's syndrome. Also makes referrals to support groups in the caller's area.

SARCOIDOSIS

National Sarcoidosis Foundation
St. Michael's Medical Center
268 Martin Luther King Blvd.
Mail Drop 73B
Newark, NJ 07102
800-223-6429
201-624-4703
24 hours a day, seven days a week

Provides information and support services to families affected by sarcoidosis. Works to increase public awareness of this condition and assists in establishing support groups.

SCOLIOSIS

Scoliosis Association
P.O. Box 811705
Boca Raton, FL 33481–1705
800-800-0669
24 hours a day, seven days a week

Provides information on scoliosis. Works to establish support networks for children and parents affected by this spinal condition. Publishes a newsletter and guidelines for starting support groups in the caller's area.

SENIOR CITIZENS' SERVICES

Alcohol Rehabilitation for the Elderly
Hopedale Medical Complex
P.O. Box 267
Hopedale, IL 61747
800-354-7089
800-344-0824 Illinois
24 hours a day, seven days a week

Provides information on treatment programs for people ages 50 and older. Also makes referrals to support groups in the caller's area.

Life Extension Foundation
995 S.W. 24th St.
Fort Lauderdale, FL 33315
800-327-6110
e-mail: LEF@lef.org

Provides information on antiaging research. Information packet available upon request.

Lighthouse National Center for Vision and Aging
111 E. 59th St.
New York, NY 10022
800-334-5497
212-808-0077
212-808-5544 TDD
9:00 A.M. to 5:00 P.M. (eastern time), Monday to Friday

Provides information to senior citizens who may be or are at risk for visual impairment. Also conducts public education programs designed for senior citizens.

National Council on the Aging
409 Third St., SW, Suite 200
Washington, DC 20024
800-424-9046
202-479-1200 District of Columbia
9:00 A.M. to 5:00 P.M. (eastern time), Monday to Friday
e-mail: info@NCOA.org

Provides general information on the subject of aging. Also serves as a clearinghouse for other organizations that provide programs to the elderly. Information packet available upon request.

National Eye Care Project Hotline
P.O. Box 429098
San Francisco, CA 94142–9098
800-222-3937
8:00 A.M. to 4:00 P.M. (Pacific time), Monday to Friday
e-mail: Tjuring@aao.org

Provides information on a program designed for people ages 65 or older who are considered economically disadvantaged. Eligibility is based on income and resources available to the person. Also makes referrals to practitioners in the caller's area.

National Institute on Aging Information Center
P.O. Box 8057
Gaithersburg, MD 20898–8057
800-222-2225
8:30 A.M. to 5:00 P.M. (eastern time), Monday to Friday
Answering machine at all other times

Provides information on all aspects of aging, especially those relating to healthy aging. Also provides information on the latest research into the biomedical, social and behavioral aspects of aging.

National Meals on Wheels Foundation
2675 44th St., SW, Suite 305
Grand Rapids, MI 49509
800-999-6262
616-531-9909
8:30 A.M. to 4:30 P.M. (central time), Monday to Friday

Provides information on the Meals on Wheels programs. Assists organizations in starting programs and recruiting volunteers. Information packet available upon request.

SEXUALLY TRANSMITTED DISEASES

STD National Hotline
American Social Health Association
P.O. Box 13827
Research Triangle Park, NC 27709
800-227-8922
919-361-8400 North Carolina
8:00 A.M. to 11:00 P.M. (eastern time), Monday to Friday

Provides confidential information on sexually transmitted diseases. Also makes referrals to practitioners in the caller's area.

SJÖGREN'S SYNDROME

National Sjögren's Syndrome Association
3201 W. Evans Dr.
Phoenix, AZ 85023
800-395-6772
602-516-0787
8:00 A.M. to 5:00 P.M. (mountain time), Monday to Friday
Answering machine at all other times
e-mail: NSSA@aol.com

Provides information on Sjögren's syndrome. Information packet, along with a list of publications, available upon request.

Sjögren's Syndrome Foundation
333 N. Broadway
Jericho, NY 11753
800-475-6473
516-933-6365
9:00 A.M. to 5:00 P.M. (eastern time), Monday to Friday
Answering machine at all other times

Provides information and educational materials. Encourages research designed to discover the causes of this condition and the development of an effective treatment. Also makes referrals to support groups in the caller's area.

SKIN DISORDERS

American Hair Loss Council
P.O. Box 809313
401 N. Michigan Ave., 22nd Floor
Chicago, IL 60606–9313
800-274-8717
312-321-5128
9:00 A.M. to 5:00 P.M. (central time), Monday to Friday
Answering machine at all other times

Provides information on the latest research into the treatment of baldness in men and women. Information packet available upon request.

American Society for Dermatological Surgery
930 N. Meacham Rd.
Schaumburg, IL 60173
800-441-2737
9:00 A.M. to 5:00 P.M. (central time), Monday to Friday
Answering machine at all other times

Provides information on surgical procedures related to skin damage from the sun, disease or aging. Also makes referrals to practitioners in the caller's area. Information packet available upon request.

National Psoriasis Foundation
6600 S.W. 92nd Ave., #300
Portland, OR 97223
800-248-0886
503-244-7404
8:00 A.M. to 5:00 P.M. (Pacific time), Monday to Friday
Answering machine at all other times
e-mail: 76135.2746@Compuserve.com

Provides information on psoriasis. Information packet available upon request.

United Scleroderma Foundation
P.O. Box 399
Watsonville, CA 95077–0399
800-722-4673
8:00 A.M. to 5:00 P.M. (Pacific time), Monday to Friday
e-mail: outreach@scleroderma.com

Provides information on scleroderma and other related skin diseases. Also makes referrals to support groups in the caller's area.

SOCIAL SECURITY

National Association of Social Security Claimants Representatives
6 Prospect St.
Midland Park, NJ 07432
800-431-2804
914-735-8812 New York (call collect)

Provides the names of attorneys who specialize in Social Security cases.

Social Security Hotline
Social Security Administration
U.S. Department of Health and Human Services
6401 Security Blvd.
Baltimore, MD 21235
800-772-1213
7:00 A.M. to 7:00 P.M. (eastern time), Monday to Friday
Answering machine at all other times

Provides information on Social Security claims and general information concerning eligibility for the program.

SPASMODIC TORTICOLLIS

National Spasmodic Torticollis Association
P.O. Box 476
Elm Grove, WI 53122–0476
800-487-8385
24 hours a day, seven days a week

Provides referrals to practitioners and support groups in the caller's area. Information packet available upon request.

SPEECH IMPAIRMENTS

American Speech-Language-Hearing Association Helpline
10801 Rockville Pike
Rockville, MD 20852
800-638-8255 Voice and TDD
800-897-8682 Alaska, Hawaii and Maryland
301-897-8682
8:30 A.M. to 4:30 P.M. (eastern time), Monday to Friday
e-mail: IRC@asha.org

Provides general information on speech, hearing and language problems. Also makes referrals to professionals in the field of speech therapy in the caller's area. Information packet available upon request.

AT&T National Special Needs Center
2001 Route 46, 3rd Floor
Parsippany, NJ 07054
800-872-3883
800-833-3232 TDD
8:30 A.M. to 6:30 P.M. (eastern time), Monday to Friday

Provides information on purchasing or renting special equipment and services available to people with hearing, speech, vision or motion impairment.

Institute of Logopedics
2400 Jardine Dr.
Wichita, KS 67219
800-835-1043 Includes Canada
800-937-4644 Canada
8:00 A.M. to 5:00 P.M. (central time), Monday to Friday

Provides information on services offered by the institute's outpatient audiology department.

National Center for Stuttering
200 E. 33rd St., Suite 17-C
New York, NY 10016
800-221-2483
9:30 A.M. to 6:00 P.M. (eastern time), Monday to Friday
e-mail: executivedirector@stuttering.com

Provides information on methods used to treat stuttering in children and adults. Information packet available upon request.

Stuttering Foundation of America
P.O. Box 11749
Memphis, TN 38111
800-992-9392
9:00 A.M. to 5:00 P.M. (central time), Monday to Friday
Answering machine at all other times

Provides information on stuttering to the public and works to assist speech pathologists in the treatment and prevention of stuttering. Also makes referrals to practitioners in the caller's area. Information packet available upon request.

Stuttering Resource Foundation
123 Oxford Rd.
New Rochelle, NY 10804
800-232-4773
914-632-3925
24 hours a day, seven days a week

Provides information on stuttering. Also makes referrals in the caller's area to speech therapists who are specialists in treating stuttering disorders. Information packet available upon request.

SPORTS MEDICINE

International Institute of Sports Science and Medicine
Center for Hip and Knee Surgery
1199 Hadley Rd.
Mooresville, IN 46158
800-237-7678 Indiana

Provides information on surgical procedures to repair hip and knee injuries.

Women's Sports Foundation
Eisenhower Park
East Meadow, NY 11554
800-227-3988
9:00 A.M. to 5:00 P.M. (eastern time), Monday to Friday
e-mail: wosport@aol.com

Provides information on women and sports, physical fitness and sports medicine. Information packet available upon request.

STROKE

AHA Stroke Connection
American Heart Association
7272 Greenville Ave.
Dallas, TX 75231
800-553-6321
214-373-6300
7:30 A.M. to 7:00 P.M. (central time), Monday to Friday
Answering machine at all other times
e-mail: strokaha@amhrt.org

Provides information on the diagnosis, treatment and prevention of stroke. Also makes referrals to support groups in the caller's area.

National Aphasia Association
P.O. Box 1887
Murray Hill Station
New York, NY 10156–0611
800-922-4622
24 hours a day, seven days a week

Provides information materials to patients and their families. Also works to raise public awareness and makes referrals to support groups in the caller's area. Information packet available upon request.

National Stroke Association
96 Inverness Dr., E, Suite 1
Englewood, CO 80112
800-787-6537
8:00 A.M. to 4:30 P.M. (mountain time), Monday to Friday

Provides information on support networks for stroke victims and their families. Also serves as a clearinghouse of information on stroke, including referrals to support groups in the caller's area.

SUBSTANCE ABUSE: ALCOHOL AND DRUGS

Al-Anon Family Group Headquarters
1600 Corporate Landing Pkwy.
Virginia Beach, VA 23454
800-356-9996
800-344-2666 Meeting information line
800-443-4525 Canada
9:00 A.M. to 5:00 P.M. (eastern time), Monday to Friday

Provides information on 12-step recovery programs for alcoholics and their families. Information packet available upon request.

Alcohol and Drug Referral Helpline
Highland Ridge Hospital
4578 S. Highland Dr.
Salt Lake City, UT 84117
800-821-4357
24 hours a day, seven days a week

Provides information on alcohol and drug abuse. Also makes referrals to support groups in the caller's area.

Alcohol Helpline
Adcare Hospital of Worcester
5 Northampton St.
Worcester, MA 01605
800-252-6465
24 hours a day, seven days a week

Provides basic information on alcohol treatment programs. Also makes referrals to treatment facilities in the caller's area.

Alcoholism and Drug Addiction Treatment Center
Scripps-Memorial Hospital
9904 Genesee Ave.
LaJolla, CA 92037
800-382-4357 California
619-457-4123

Provides information on substance abuse treatment programs. Also makes referrals to treatment services for adults and adolescents.

American Council for Drug Education
164 W. 74th St.
New York, NY 10023
800-488-3784
800-262-2463 Cocaine hotline
212-595-5810
24 hours a day, seven days a week

Provides information and referrals to drug rehabilitation programs in the caller's area. Also answers specific questions on substance abuse.

American Council on Alcoholism
2522 St. Paul St.
Baltimore, MD 21218
800-527-5344
410-889-0100 Baltimore
9:00 A.M. to 5:00 P.M. (eastern time), Monday to Friday
Answering machine at all other times

Provides information on alcoholism prevention programs for adults and children. Also provides counseling and referrals to treatment programs in the caller's area.

ASAP Treatment Hotline
P.O. Box 6150
Malibu, CA 90264
800-367-2727

Provides counseling and information on substance abuse treatment programs in the caller's area. Information packet available upon request.

BABES World
Beginning Alcohol and Addiction Basic Education Studies
33 E. Forest St.
Detroit, MI 48201
800-542-2237

Provides information on alcohol and drug prevention programs designed for children. Information packet available upon request.

Cocaine Anonymous
3740 Overland Ave., Suite G
Los Angeles, CA 90034
800-347-8998
310-559-5833 Los Angeles
24 hours a day, seven days a week

Provides information on cocaine addiction and rehabilitation programs. Information packet available upon request.

Cottage Program International
75 E. Fort Union Blvd.
Midvale, UT 84047
800-752-6100
24 hours a day, seven days a week

Provides information on substance abuse treatment programs for families. Also makes referrals to chapters in the caller's area. Information packet available upon request.

Drug Abuse Information and Treatment Referral Line
National Institute on Drug Abuse
11426 Rockville Pike, Suite 410
Rockville, MD 20852
800-662-4357
800-662-9832 Spanish
800-228-0427 TDD
9:00 A.M. to 3:00 P.M. (eastern time), Monday to Friday
Noon to 3:00 P.M. (eastern time), Saturday and Sunday
Answering machine at all other times

Provides counseling and referral services to callers. Also provides general information on substance abuse and addiction. Information packet available upon request.

Drug Abuse Resistance Education (DARE)
P.O. Box 512090
Los Angeles, CA 90051–0090
800-223-3273

Provides information on programs that teach people how to avoid using drugs and other harmful substances. Information packet available upon request.

Families Anonymous
P.O. Box 3475
Culver City, CA 90231
800-736-9805
818-989-7841
e-mail: famanon@earthlink.net

Provides information for families with children who have substance abuse or behavioral problems. Also provides counseling for family members and friends.

Family Talk About Drinking
Anheuser-Busch Company
Department of Consumer Awareness and Education
1 Busch Pl.
St. Louis, MO 63118
800-359-8255
9:00 A.M. to 5:00 P.M. (central time), Monday to Friday
Answering machine at all other times

Provides information to families on how to discuss alcohol use with young children and teenagers. Message also available in Spanish. Information packet available upon request.

Hazelton Foundation
15251 Pleasant Valley Rd.
P.O. Box 176
Center City, MN 55012
800-328-9000
800-262-5010 Minnesota
7:00 A.M. to 6:00 P.M. (central time), Monday to Friday
Answering machine at all other times

Provides information on substance abuse treatment and rehabilitation programs. Operates a rehabilitation center. Also makes referrals to other organizations and resources in the caller's area. Information packet available upon request.

Johnson Institute
7205 Ohms Ln., Suite 200
Minneapolis, MN 55439–2159
800-231-5165
800-247-0484 Minnesota
e-mail: info@Johnsoninstitute.com

Provides educational materials and information on community substance abuse prevention programs in the caller's area.

Mothers Against Drunk Drivers (MADD)
511 E. John Carpenter Freeway, Suite 700
Irving, TX 75062
800-438-6233
24 hours a day, seven days a week

Provides information on programs designed to prevent drunk driving. Information packet available upon request.

National Clearinghouse for Alcohol and Drug Information
11426-28 Rockville Pike, Suite 200
Rockville, MD 20852
800-729-6686
8:00 A.M. to 5:00 P.M. (eastern time), Monday to Friday
e-mail: info@health.org

Provides information and referrals to callers with questions about alcohol and drug treatment programs in the caller's area. Information packet available upon request.

National Council on Alcoholism and Drug Dependence Hopeline
12 W. 21st St.
New York, NY 10010
800-622-2255
212-206-6770 New York City
24 hours a day, seven days a week

Provides information on rehabilitation programs. Also makes referrals to support groups in the caller's area. Information packet available upon request.

National Parents Resources Institute for Drug Education
3610 Dekalb Technology Pkwy., Suite 105
Atlanta, GA 30340
800-853-7867
404-577-4500 Atlanta
e-mail: PRC@MINDSPRING.Com

Provides information on how to start community drug education programs for young people. Information packet available upon request.

New Life (Women for Sobriety)
P.O. Box 618
Quakertown, PA 18951
800-333-1606
215-536-8026

Provides assistance to women alcoholics. Information packet available upon request.

Pride Institute
101 Fifth Ave.
New York, NY 10003
800-547-7433
24 hours a day, seven days a week

Provides information for persons addicted to alcohol or drugs. Also makes referrals to treatment centers in the caller's area.

SUDDEN INFANT DEATH SYNDROME

American Sudden Infant Death Syndrome Institute
6065 Roswell Rd., Suite 876
Atlanta, GA 30328
800-232-7437
800-847-7437 Georgia
8:00 A.M. to 5:00 P.M. (eastern time), Monday to Friday
Answering machine at all other times
e-mail: parent@sids.org

Provides information on the latest research into the causes of sudden infant death syndrome. Also provides counseling and makes referrals to support groups in the caller's area. Information packet available upon request.

Sudden Infant Death Syndrome Alliance
1314 Bedford Ave., Suite 210
Baltimore, MD 21208
800-221-7437
9:00 A.M. to 5:00 P.M. (eastern time), Monday to Friday
Answering machine at all other times

Provides information to parents of young infants. Also offers counseling and support services to parents who have lost a child to sudden infant death syndrome. Information packet available upon request.

SURGERY SERVICES

American Academy of Facial Plastic and Reconstructive Surgery
1110 Vermont Ave., NW, Suite 220
Washington, DC 20005
800-332-3223
800-532-3223 Canada
202-842-4500 District of Columbia
24 hours a day, seven days a week

Provides general information on plastic surgery. Also makes referrals to practitioners in the caller's area.

American Association of Oral and Maxillofacial Surgeons
9700 Bryn Mawr Ave.
Rosemont, IL 60018
800-467-5268
8:30 A.M. to 5:00 P.M. (central time), Monday to Friday
Answering machine at all other times

Provides information on temporomandibular joint and other jaw disorders, as well as oral cancer. Also makes referrals to practitioners in the caller's area. Information packet available upon request.

American Plastic Surgery Information
6707 First Ave., S
St. Petersburg, FL 33707
800-522-2222 Florida

Provides information on plastic and reconstructive surgery. Also makes referrals to practitioners in the caller's area. Information packet available upon request.

American Society of Plastic and Reconstructive Surgeons
444 E. Algonquin Rd.
Arlington Heights, IL 60005
800-635-0635
8:30 A.M. to 4:30 P.M. (central time), Monday to Friday
Answering machine at all other times

Provides information on surgical procedures. Also makes referrals to practitioners in the caller's area and verifies credentials of plastic surgeons. Information packet available upon request.

Plastic and Aesthetic Surgery Center
217 E. Chestnut St.
Louisville, KY 40202
800-327-3613
800-633-8923 Kentucky
24 hours a day, seven days a week

Provides information on various plastic surgery procedures, including cost estimates. Also makes referrals to practitioners in the caller's area.

SYRINGOMYELIA

American Syringomyelia Alliance Project
P.O. Box 1586
Longview, TX 75606–1586
800-ASAP-282 (800-272-7282)
903-236-7079
24 hours a day, seven days a week

Provides information and support to patients and their families. Also makes referrals to support groups in the caller's area. Sponsors an annual conference.

TOURETTE SYNDROME

Tourette Syndrome Association
42-40 Bell Blvd.
Bayside, NY 11361
800-237-0717
9:00 A.M. to 5:00 P.M. (eastern time), Monday to Friday
Answering machine at all other times
e-mail: tourette@ix.netcom.com

Provides information on Tourette syndrome to patients and their families. Also makes referrals to chapters in the caller's area.

TOXIC SUBSTANCES

Asbestos Technical Information Service
P.O. Box 12194
Research Triangle Park, NC 27709
800-334-8571
9:00 A.M. to 5:00 P.M. (eastern time), Monday to Friday

Provides information on different types of asbestos and proper removal and disposal procedures. Also provides information on home tests for asbestos. Information packet available upon request.

Chemical Manufacturers Association
1300 Wilson Blvd.
Arlington, VA 22209
800-262-8200
202-887-1315 District of Columbia
9:00 A.M. to 6:00 P.M. (eastern time), Monday to Friday
Answering machine at all other times
e-mail: chemtrec@mail.cmahq.com

Provides general information on the safe handling of chemicals. Also makes referrals to the manufacturers of specific chemical products who are responsible for providing more detailed information on the proper use of their products. Information packet available upon request.

Emergency Planning and Community Right-to-Know Information Hotline
U.S. Environmental Protection Agency
401 M St., NW
Washington, DC 20460
800-535-0202
202-479-2449 District of Columbia
9:00 A.M. to 6:00 P.M. (eastern time), Monday to Friday
Answering machine at all other times

Provides information on the types of chemicals that are stored and used in the community and workplace. Also provides information on the requirements of the Emergency Planning and Community Right-to-Know Act of 1986.

Environmental Defense Fund Hotline
1616 P St., NW
Washington, DC 20036
800-225-5333
202-387-3500 District of Columbia
9:00 A.M. to 5:00 P.M. (eastern time), Monday to Friday

Provides information to the public on the issue of environmental protection, including ways in which individuals can help keep the environment clean. Information packet available upon request.

National Center for Toxicological Research
3900 NCTR Rd.
Jefferson, AR 72079–9502
800-638-3321
9:00 A.M. to 5:00 P.M. (central time), Monday to Friday

Provides information on the effects of toxic substances on the environment.

TUBEROUS SCLEROSIS

National Tuberous Sclerosis Association
8181 Professional Pl., Suite 110
Landover, MD 20785
800-225-6872
301-459-9888 Maryland
9:00 A.M. to 5:00 P.M. (eastern time), Monday to Friday
Answering machine at all other times
e-mail: ntsa@aol.com

Provides referrals to representatives of the association. Also provides information on parent-to-parent support networks in the caller's area. Information packet available upon request.

UROLOGIC DISEASES

American Foundation for Urologic Disease
300 W. Pratt St., Suite 401
Baltimore, MD 21201
800-242-2383
410-727-2908
8:00 A.M. to 10:00 P.M. (eastern time), Monday to Friday

Provides information on the various types of adult and pediatric urologic diseases. Promotes research and conducts education programs to raise the public awareness on these conditions. Sponsors the Us Too prostate cancer survivors program. Information packet available upon request.

VIETNAM VETERANS

Vietnam Veterans Agent Orange Victims
P.O. Box 2465
Darien, CT 06820–0465
800-521-0198
9:00 A.M. to 4:00 P.M. (eastern time), Monday to Friday
Answering machine at all other times

Provides medical and legal advice, information and counseling to veterans who have been exposed to the defoliant Agent Orange. Operates a children's fund to aid families whose children may be suffering from birth defects and developmental disabilities linked to Agent Orange. Information packet available upon request.

VISION IMPAIRMENTS

See also: **RETINITIS PIGMENTOSA**

American Council of the Blind
1155 15th St., NW, Suite 1155
Washington, DC 20005
800-424-8666
202-467-5081 District of Columbia
3:00 P.M. to 5:30 P.M. (eastern time), Monday to Friday
e-mail: ncrabb@access.digex.net

Provides information and referrals to clinics, organizations and government agencies that provide services to the blind. Information packet available upon request.

American Foundation for the Blind
11 Pennsylvania Ave., Suite 300
New York, NY 10001
800-232-5463
212-502-7662 TDD
8:30 A.M. to 4:30 P.M. (eastern time), Monday to Friday
e-mail: afbinfo@abf.org

Provides answers to questions concerning vision loss and blindness. Information packet available upon request.

American Printing House for the Blind
1839 Frankfort Ave.
P.O. Box 6085
Louisville, KY 40206–6085
800-223-1839
502-895-2405

Provides information on braille, large-type books and computer disks for visually impaired persons. Information packet and catalog available upon request.

AT&T National Special Needs Center
2001 Route 46, 3rd Floor
Parsippany, NJ 07054
800-872-3883
800-833-3232 TDD
8:30 A.M. to 6:30 P.M. (eastern time), Monday to Friday

Provides information on purchasing or renting special equipment and services available to people with hearing, speech, vision or motion impairment.

Audio Reader
P.O. Box 847
Lawrence, KS 66044
800-772-8898 Kansas

Provides information on reading services available to visually impaired persons.

Blind Children's Center
4120 Marathon St.
Los Angeles, CA 90029–0159
800-222-3566
800-222-3567 California
e-mail: info@blindcntr.org

Provides information on blindness. Also makes referrals to organizations and support groups in the caller's area.

Books on Tape
P.O. Box 7900
Newport Beach, CA 92658–7900
800-626-3333

Provides information on how to obtain books on tape for visually impaired persons. Information packet available upon request.

Guide Dog Foundation for the Blind
371 E. Jericho Turnpike
Smithtown, NY 11787
800-548-4337
9:00 A.M. to 5:00 P.M. (eastern time), Monday to Friday
e-mail: guidedog@guidedog.org

Provides information on the guide dog program. Also makes referrals to support groups in the caller's area.

Job Opportunities for the Blind
1800 Johnson St.
Baltimore, MD 21230
800-638-7518
12:30 P.M. to 5:00 P.M. (eastern time), Monday to Friday

Provides career counseling, job listings and referrals to visually impaired persons who are seeking employment.

National Service for the Blind and Physically Handicapped
National Library of Congress
1291 Taylor St., NW
Washington, DC 20542
800-424-8567
202-794-8650 District of Columbia
8:00 A.M. to 4:30 P.M. (eastern time), Monday to Thursday
e-mail: nls@loc.gov

Provides information on libraries that offer books on audiotape and books in braille.

National Society to Prevent Blindness
National Center for Sight
500 E. Remington Rd., Suite 200
Schaumberg, IL 60173
800-221-3004
8:00 A.M. to 5:00 P.M. (central time), Monday to Friday
e-mail: 7477.100@Compuserve.com

Provides literature on specific vision problems and conditions. Also produces educational materials and offers professional education programs. Information packet available upon request.

Recording for the Blind
20 Roszel Rd.
Princeton, NJ 08540
800-221-4792
609-452-0606
9:00 A.M. to 9:00 P.M. (eastern time), Monday to Friday
Answering machine at all other times

Provides information on how to obtain recordings for visually impaired persons. Information packet available upon request.

WOMEN'S HEALTH

See also: **PREGNANCY SERVICES; PREMENSTRUAL SYNDROME**

Breast Implant Information Service
Food and Drug Administration
P.O. Box 1802
Rockville, MD 20704–1802
800-532-4440
800-688-6167 TDD
10:00 A.M. to 4:00 P.M. (eastern time), Monday to Friday
Answering machine at all other times

Provides information on the status of clinical studies being conducted on the safety of silicone-gel-filled breast implants. Information packet available upon request.

DES Action
1615 Broadway, Suite 510
Oakland, CA 94612
800-337-9288
510-465-4011

Provides information on the effects of DES (diethylstilbestrol) on the children of mothers who took the medication while pregnant. Promotes public awareness and offers support to DES-affected daughters and sons. Information packet available upon request.

Johnson and Johnson
Personal Products Consumer Response Center
New Brunswick, NJ 08901
800-526-3967

Provides information on a wide range of women's health concerns, including toxic shock syndrome.

Planned Parenthood Federation of America
810 Seventh Ave.
New York, NY 10019
800-829-7732
8:30 A.M. to 5:00 P.M. (eastern time), Monday to Friday

Provides information on a wide range of women's health issues, including general health and wellness, family planning, patient education and abortion. Also makes referrals to Planned Parenthood clinics in the caller's area.

Women's Sports Foundation
Eisenhower Park
East Meadow, NY 11554
800-227-3988
9:00 A.M. to 5:00 P.M. (eastern time), Monday to Friday
e-mail: wosport@aol.com

Provides information on women and sports, physical fitness and sports medicine. Information packet available upon request.

DIAL 800 FOR HEALTH INDEX AND SUBJECT CROSS-REFERENCE

A

B

C

D

E

F

G

H

I

J

K

L

S

T

U

V

W